Mpho's Legacy of Hope
Coloring Book

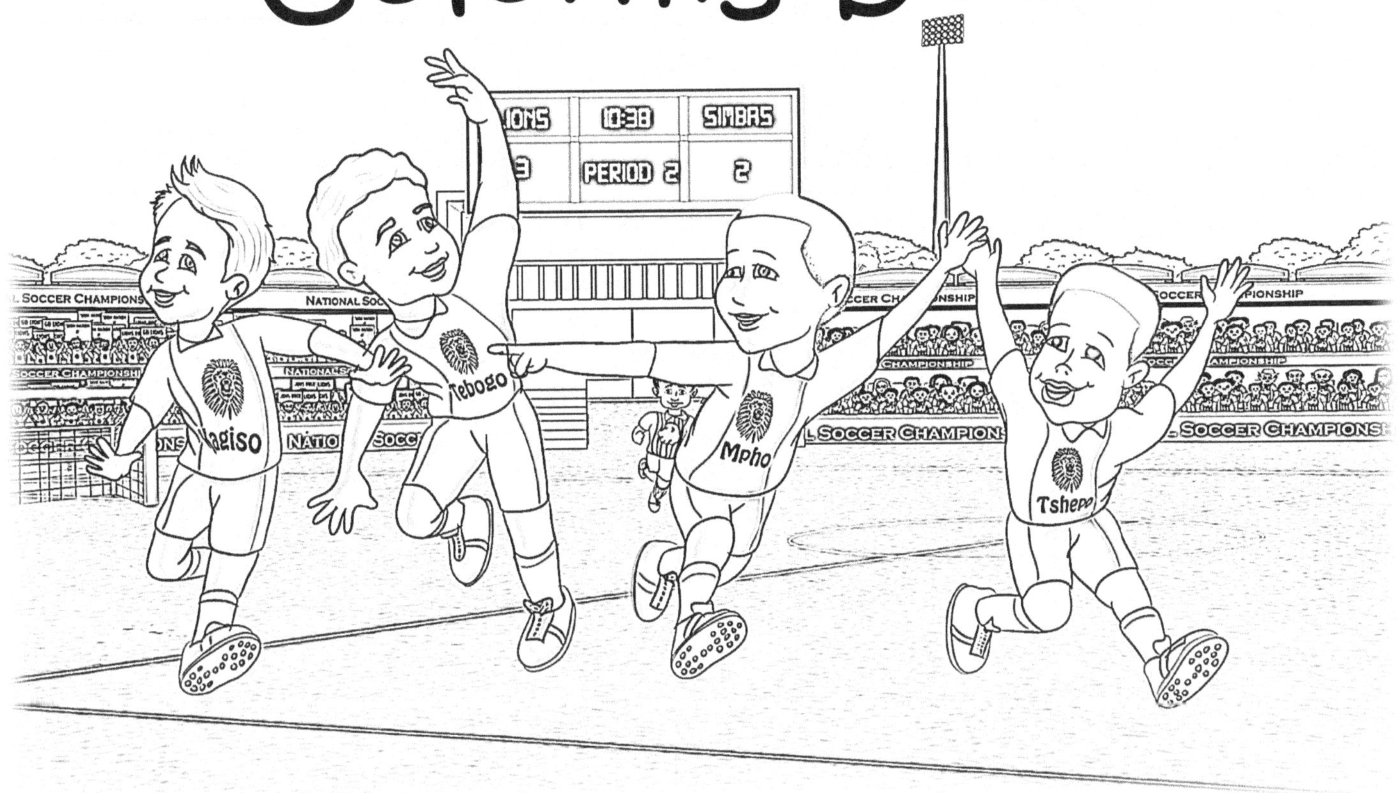

An Inspired Story of Living With HIV/AIDS

Written By:

Dr. Wyntrea Cunningham

Whitehall Publishing
PO Box 548
Yellville, AR 72687
info@whitehallpublishing.com
http://whitehallpublishing.com

The Hope Ambassador Doll
on the Front Cover

The Hope Ambassador Doll Project is an art therapy program, using dolls, to help reduce the fear and anxiety that children encounter as a result of either being infected by, or impacted by HIV/AIDS. The doll itself is appropriately called Hope, and children can paint faces on their Hope doll and include encouraging messages as well. The dolls can then be exchanged with other children whose lives have been affected by HIV/AIDS around the world. The original Hope doll was created by a child who was infected with HIV/AIDS. She (Hope) acts as the ambassador for the project, spreading the message, "I know there is Hope, because I have seen her with my own eyes.

Retail Price: $9.95
Printed in the U.S.A.

Preface

In 2003 I had a wonderful opportunity to spend three months in Gaborone, Botswana (Hah-ba-ronay, Bots-wana) conducting research with the Baylor International Pediatric AIDS Initiative (BIPAI). Having done some HIV/AIDS research in college, I became aware of the impact of the stigma surrounding the disease, and I really wanted to help. I decided to write a children's book to address and dispel some of the myths surrounding HIV/AIDS in order to help decrease the stigma associated with it. Additionally, this book conveys a message of hope that HIV is no longer a death sentence, and it also serves to encourage more conversations about HIV, and in doing so we are educating more people about the disease. The importance of this book and further research in reducing the stigma of HIV/AIDS was so eloquently stated by Dr. Cathy Wilfert, a pioneer in helping to reduce mother to child transmission of HIV, when she stated,

"Children make up 30% of our world's population,
but they are 100% of our future."

The main characters in this book were given Setswanan (Sets-swah-nan) names for the native language spoken in Gaborone, with the following meanings:

Mpho (Mm-poh)   = gift,
Kagiso (Kah-heeso)= peace,
Tshepo (Sheh-poh) = hope & trust,
Tebogo (Teh-bogo) = we are thankful.

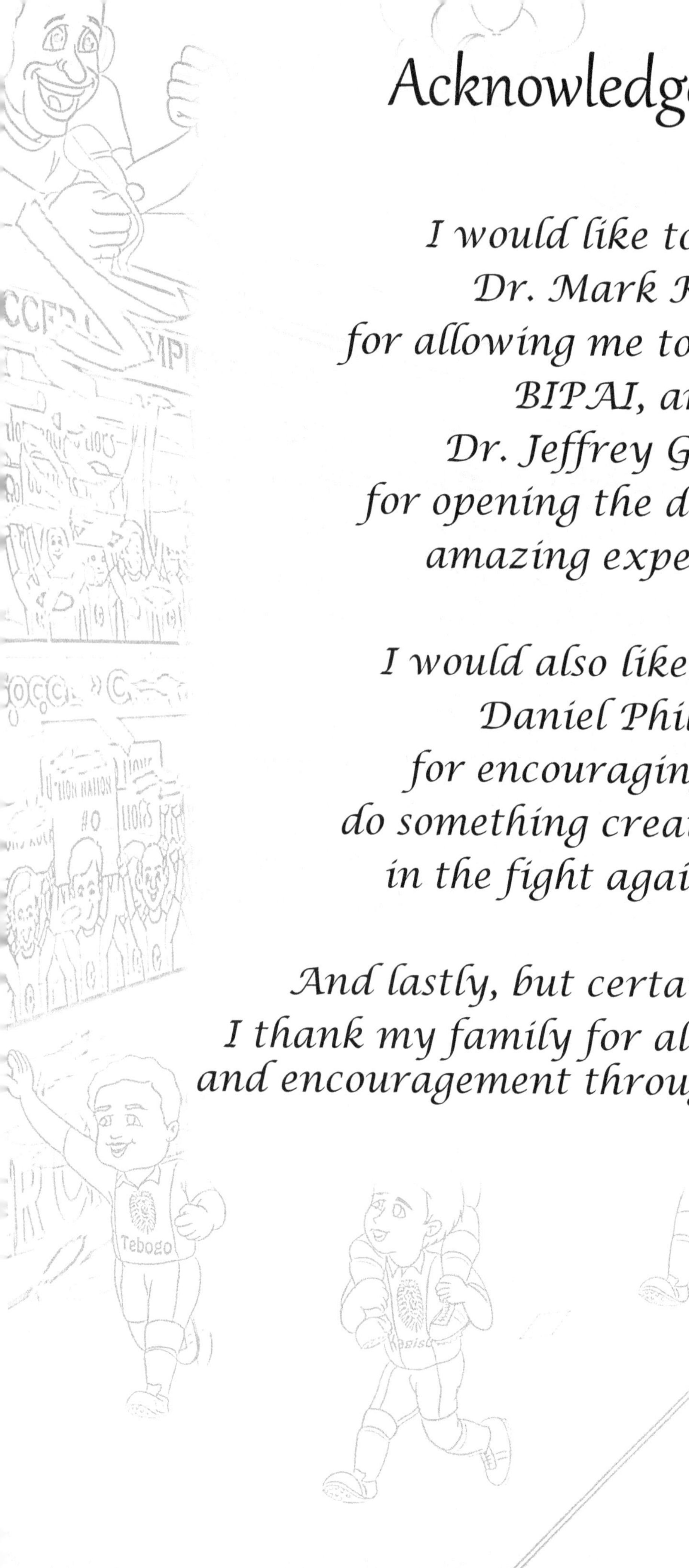

Acknowledgements

I would like to thank
Dr. Mark Kline
for allowing me to work with
BIPAI, and
Dr. Jeffrey Guidry
for opening the door to this
amazing experience.

I would also like to thank
Daniel Phillips
for encouraging me to
do something creative to help
in the fight against HIV.

And lastly, but certainly not least,
I thank my family for all of their support
and encouragement throughout my journey.

Dedication

To my parents:

*Words cannot express
how truly grateful I am
to have such wonderful parents
and how much I appreciate your
sacrifices in helping me
reach my dreams.*

Thank you for everything!

"Listen up guys, it's halftime,
the score is tied at two. You have all worked
hard and I know we can win this thing.

Tshepo, Kagiso, Tebogo I want you to get the
ball to Mpho so he can work his magic."
The coach said.

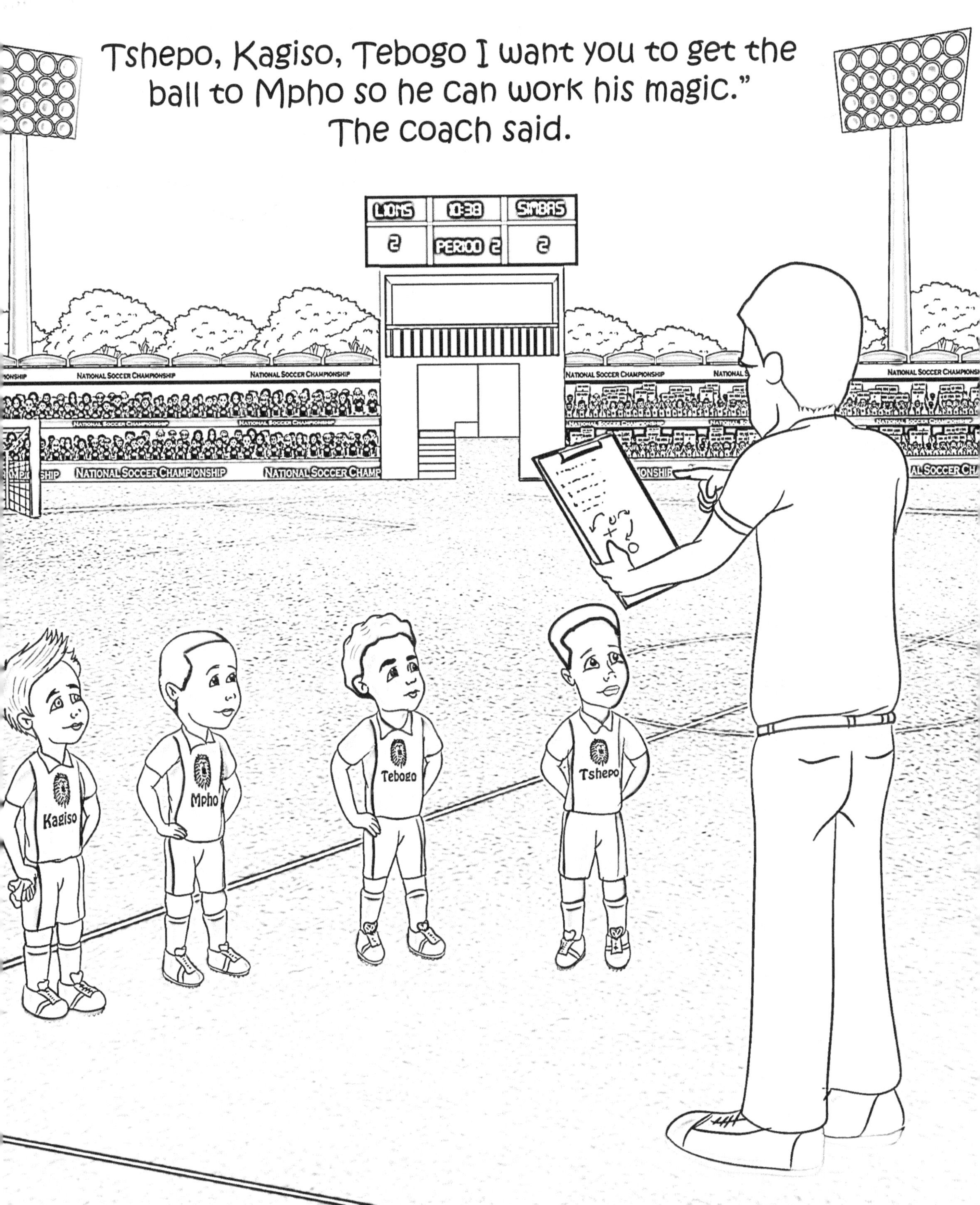

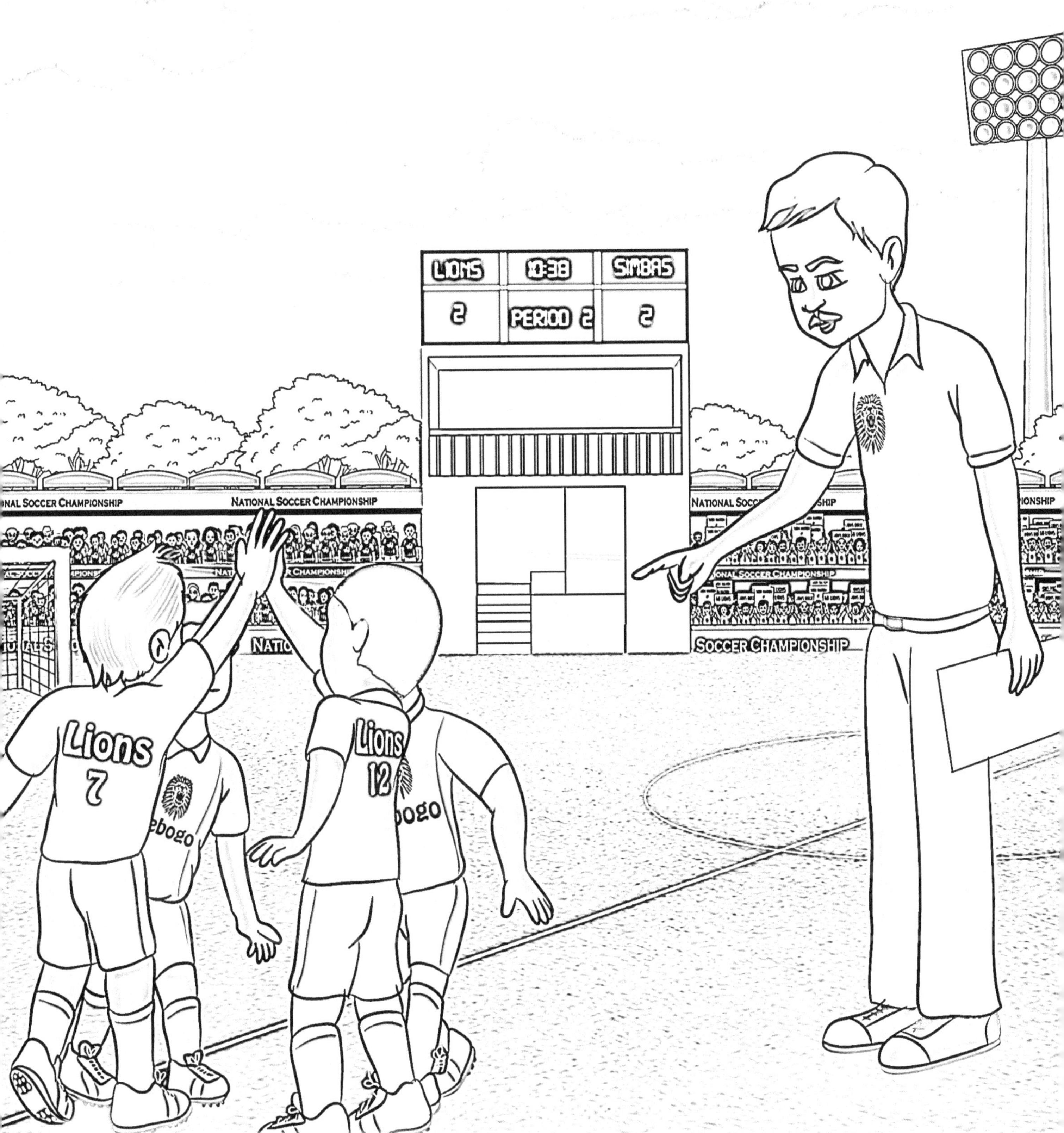

"Mpho, I want you to do your thing and score.
Remember, ignore the screaming crowds,
concentrate and focus, then you can do it.
Alright team on 3, 1-2-3 Let's Win!"
The coach said.

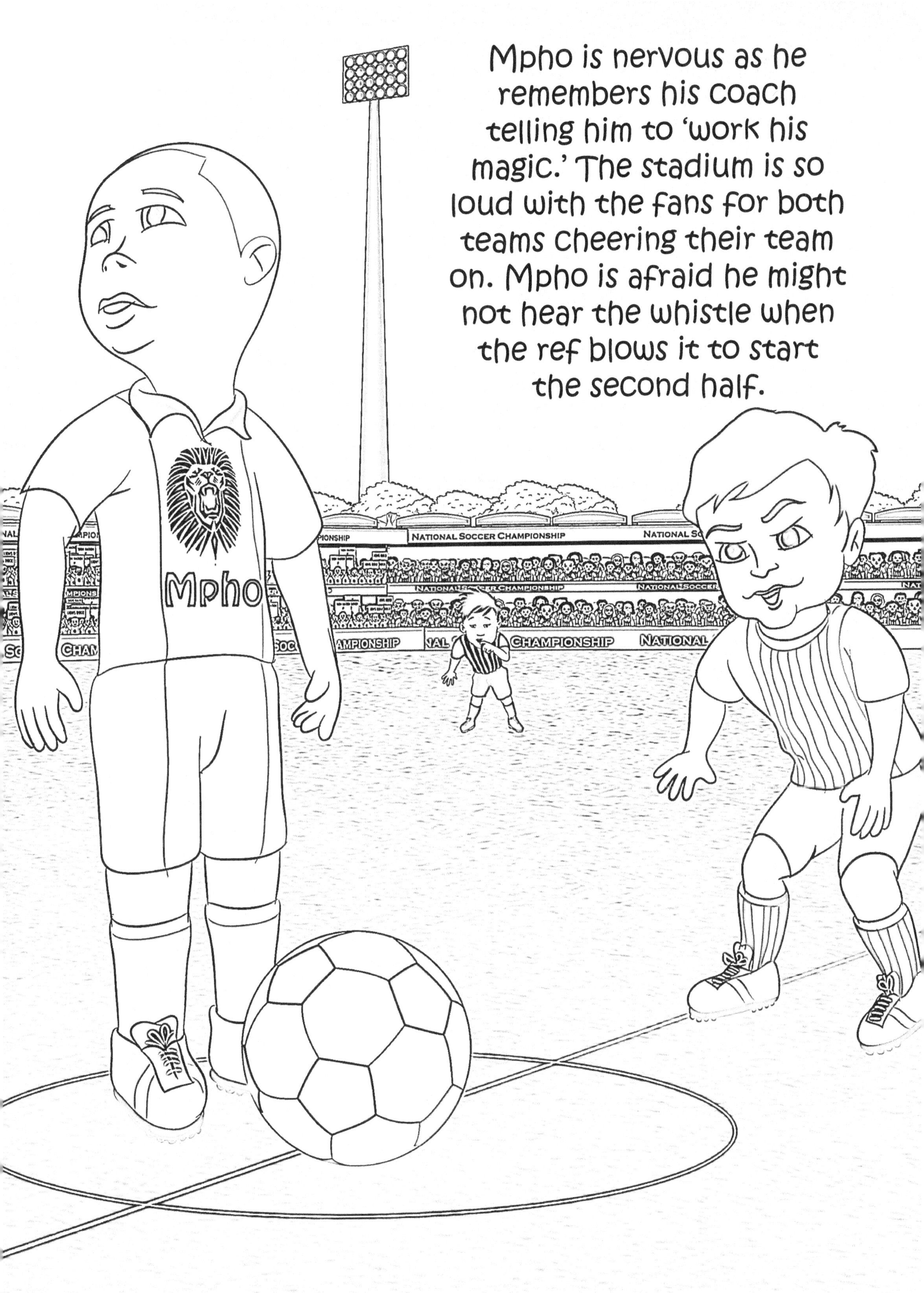

Mpho is nervous as he remembers his coach telling him to 'work his magic.' The stadium is so loud with the fans for both teams cheering their team on. Mpho is afraid he might not hear the whistle when the ref blows it to start the second half.
Mpho
NATIONAL SOCCER CHAMPIONSHIP

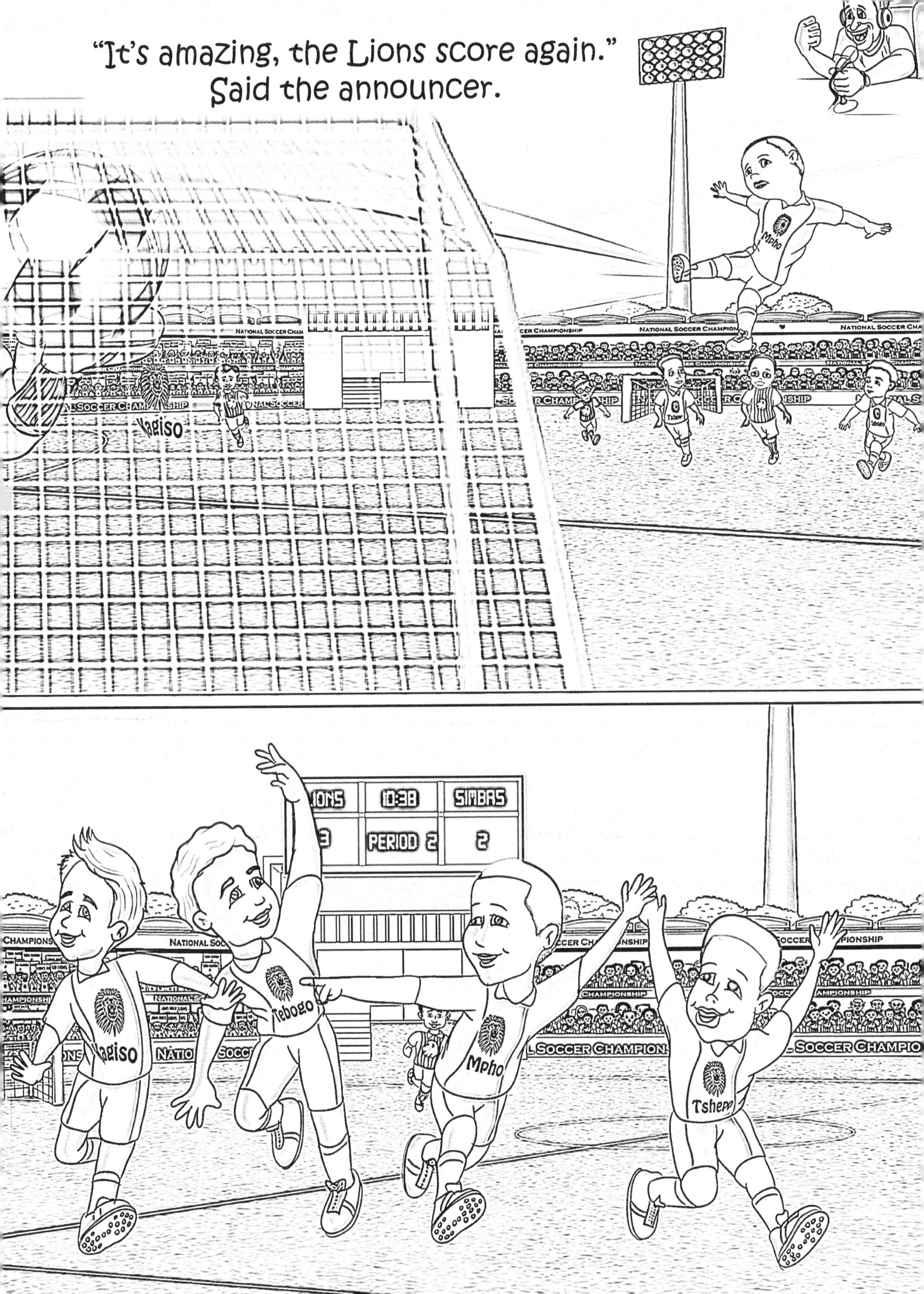

"It's amazing, the Lions score again."
Said the announcer.
Nagiso
National Soccer Championship
Tshepo
Mpho
LIONS 10:38 SIMBAS
3 PERIOD 2 2
Nagiso
Tebogo
Mpho
Tshepo

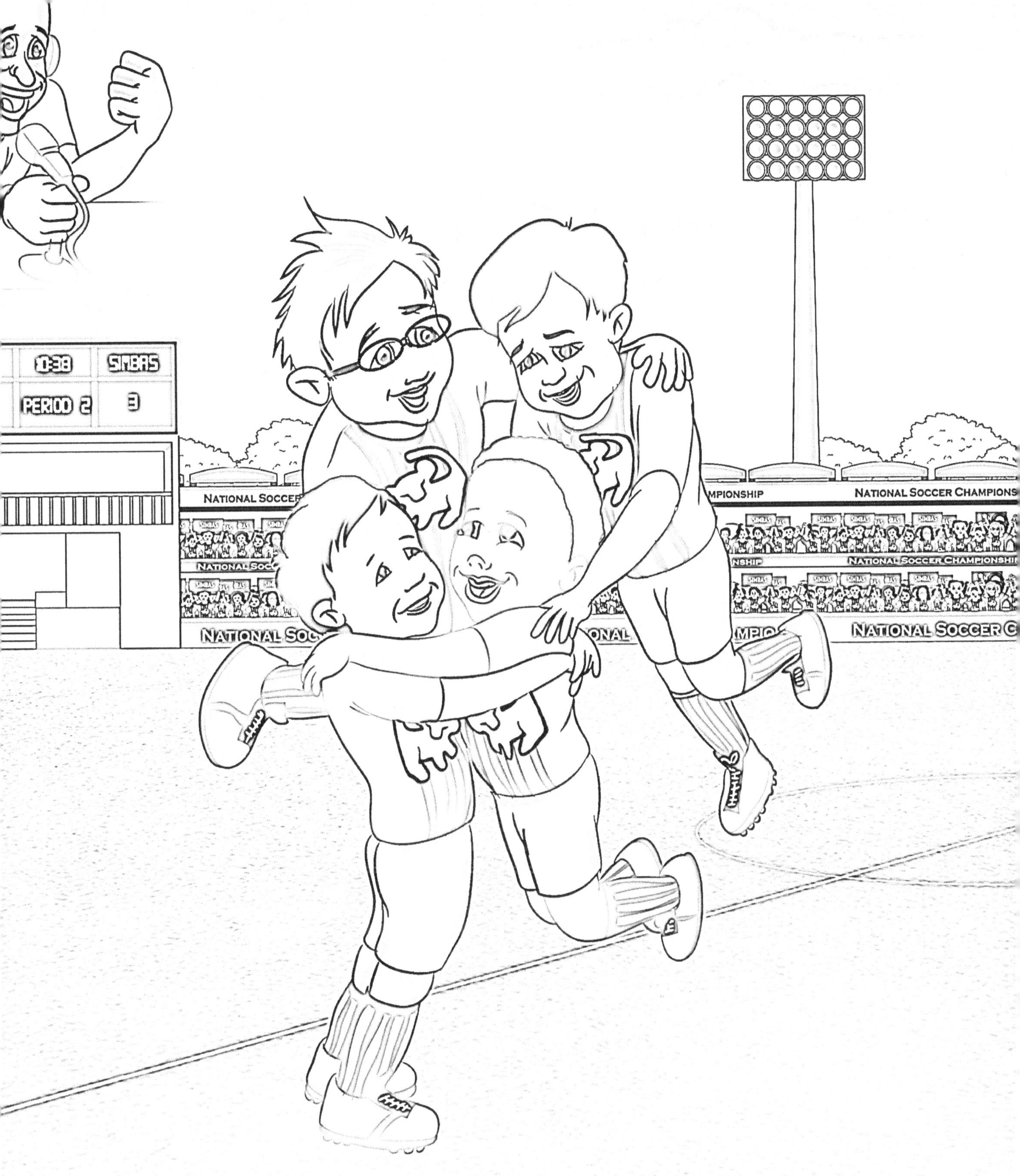

"But wait, with only minutes left to play, the Simbas score again! The big championship game is all tied up at 3-3." The announcer shouted as the crowd erupted with excitement.

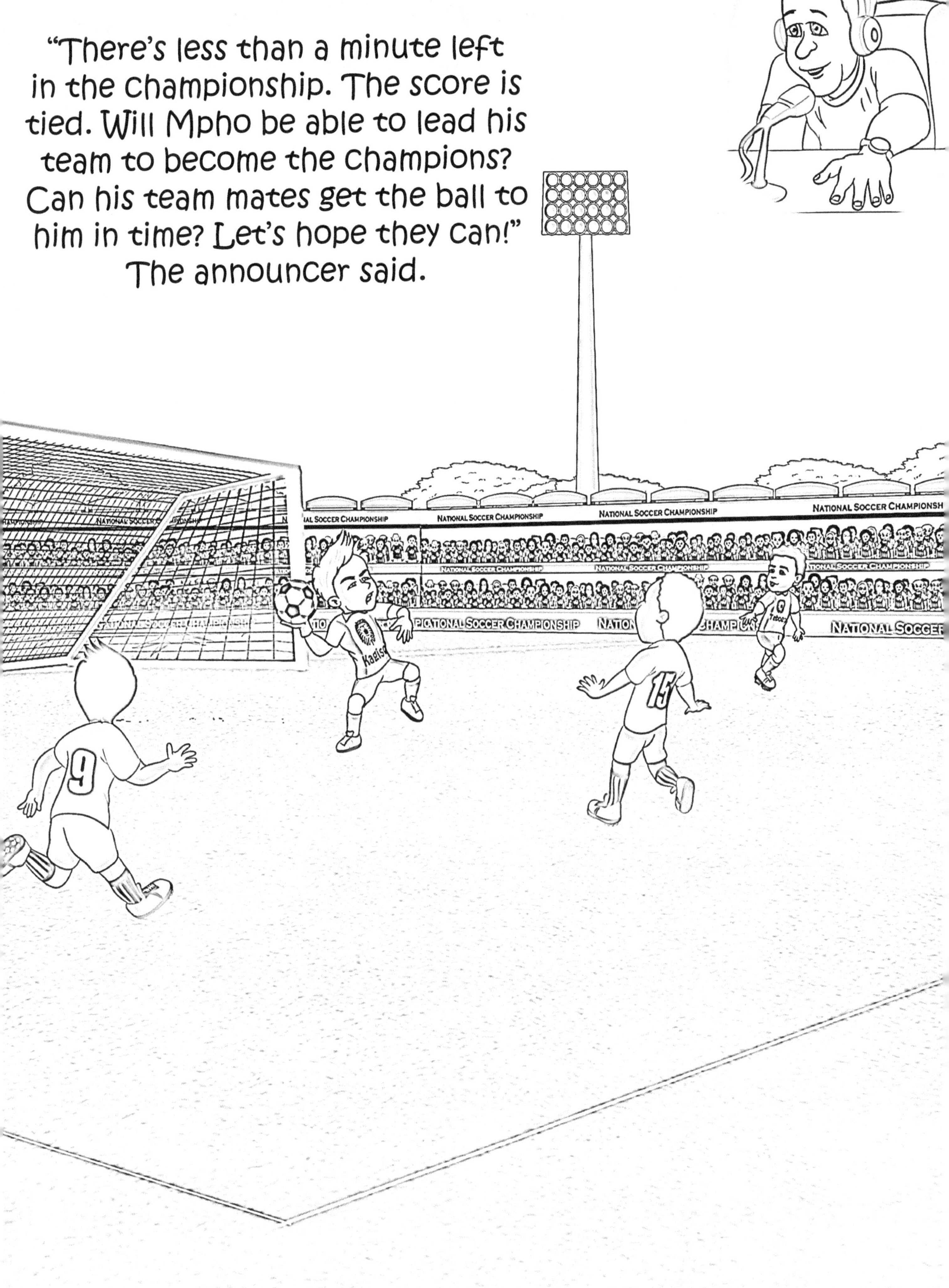

"There's less than a minute left in the championship. The score is tied. Will Mpho be able to lead his team to become the champions? Can his team mates get the ball to him in time? Let's hope they can!" The announcer said.

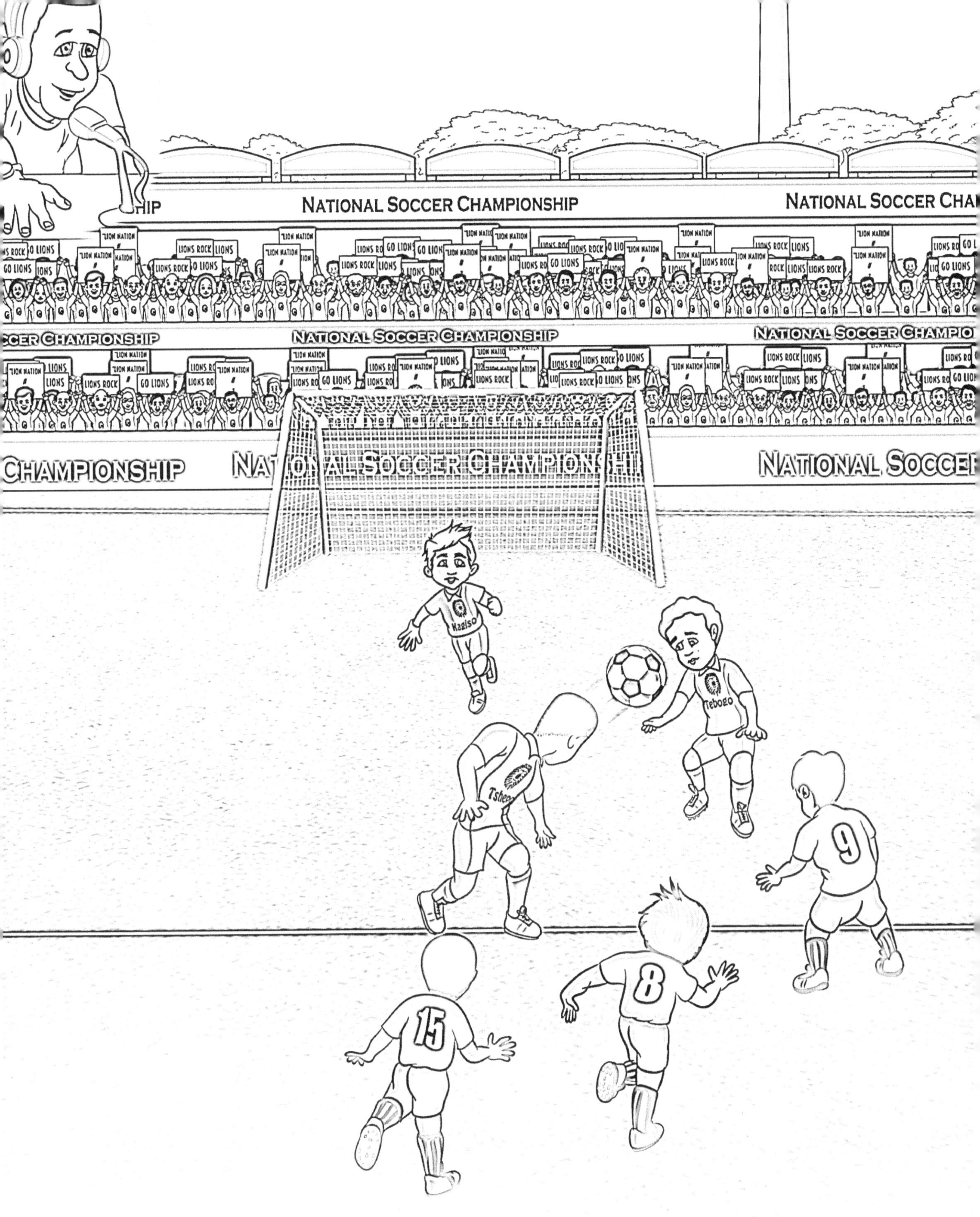

"Kagiso passes the ball to Tshepo who head butts the ball to Tebogo." The announcer exclaimed with excitement.

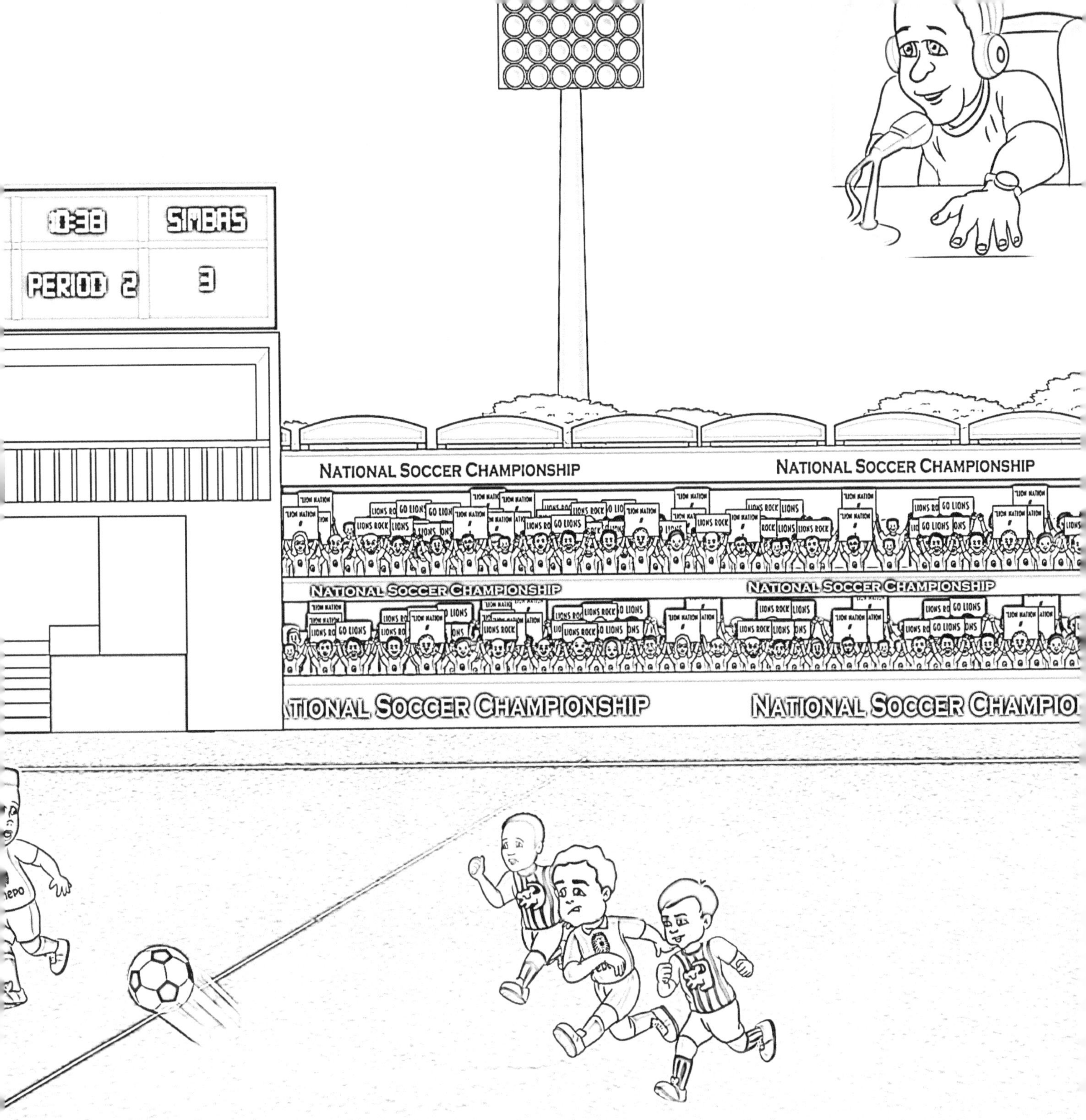

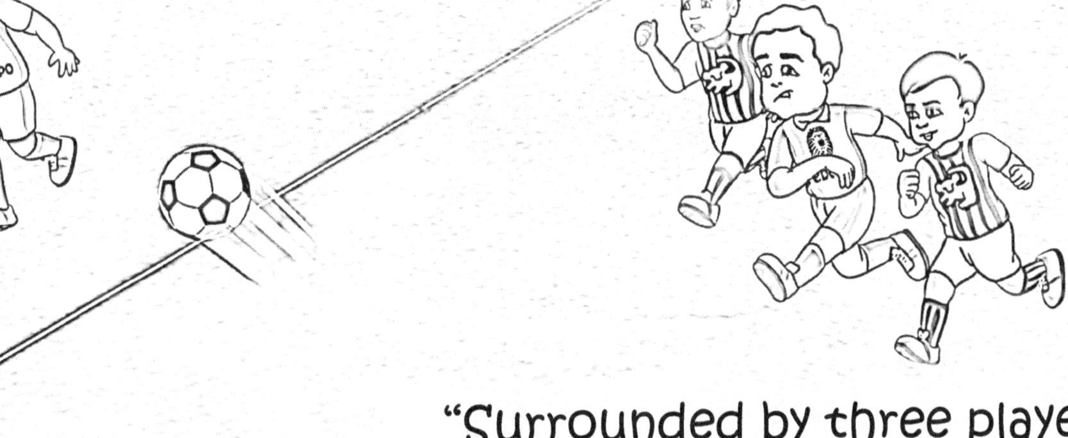

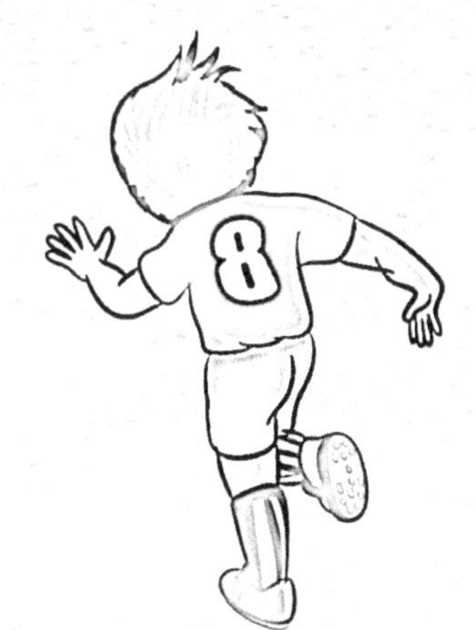

"Surrounded by three players from the other team, Tebogo is trapped. But wait, he kicks the ball into an open space near middle of the field. There are only seconds remaining in this championship contest. Will Mpho's teammates be able to get the ball to him in time and if they do, will he be able to score?" The announcer shouts.

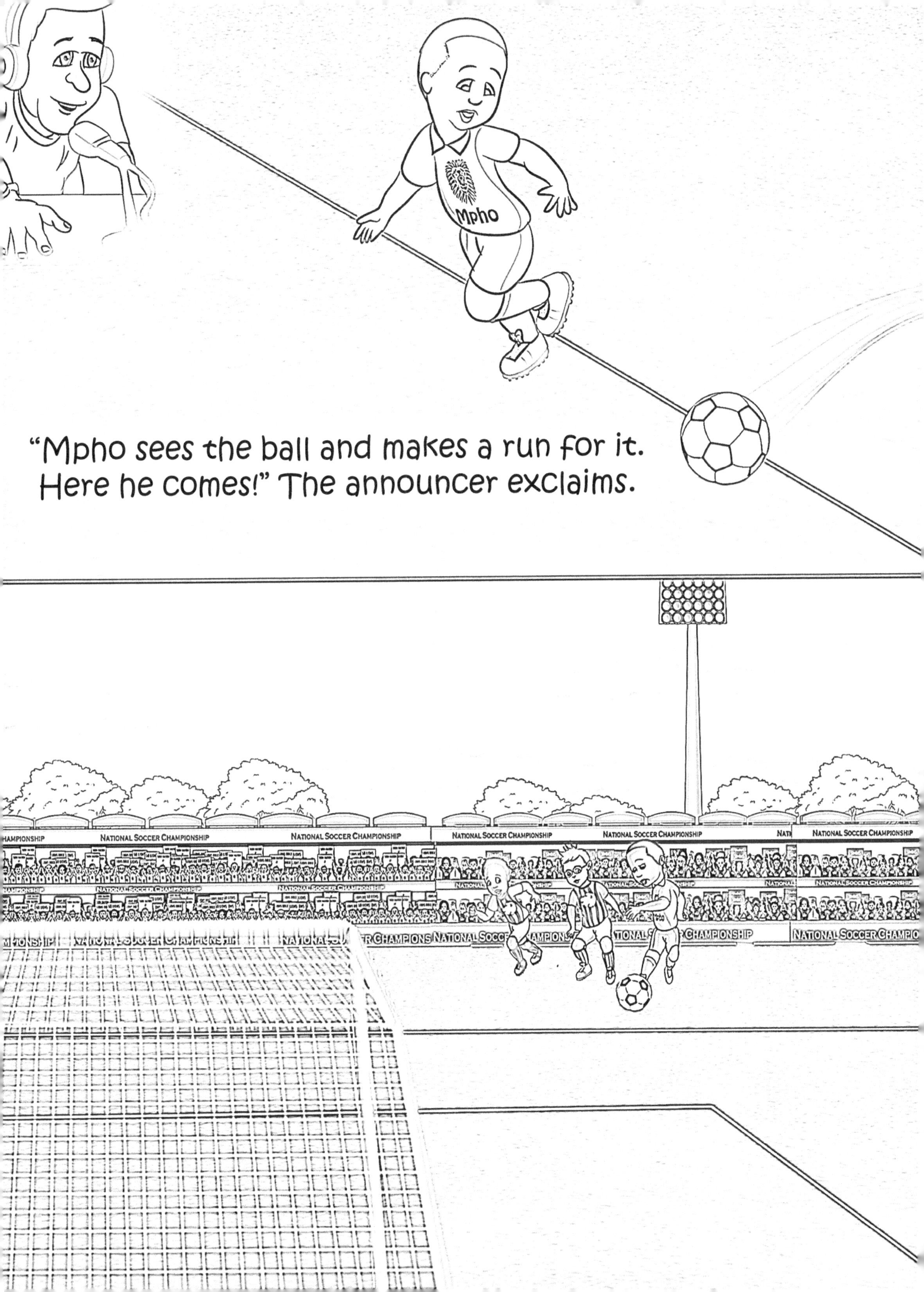

"Mpho sees the ball and makes a run for it. Here he comes!" The announcer exclaims.

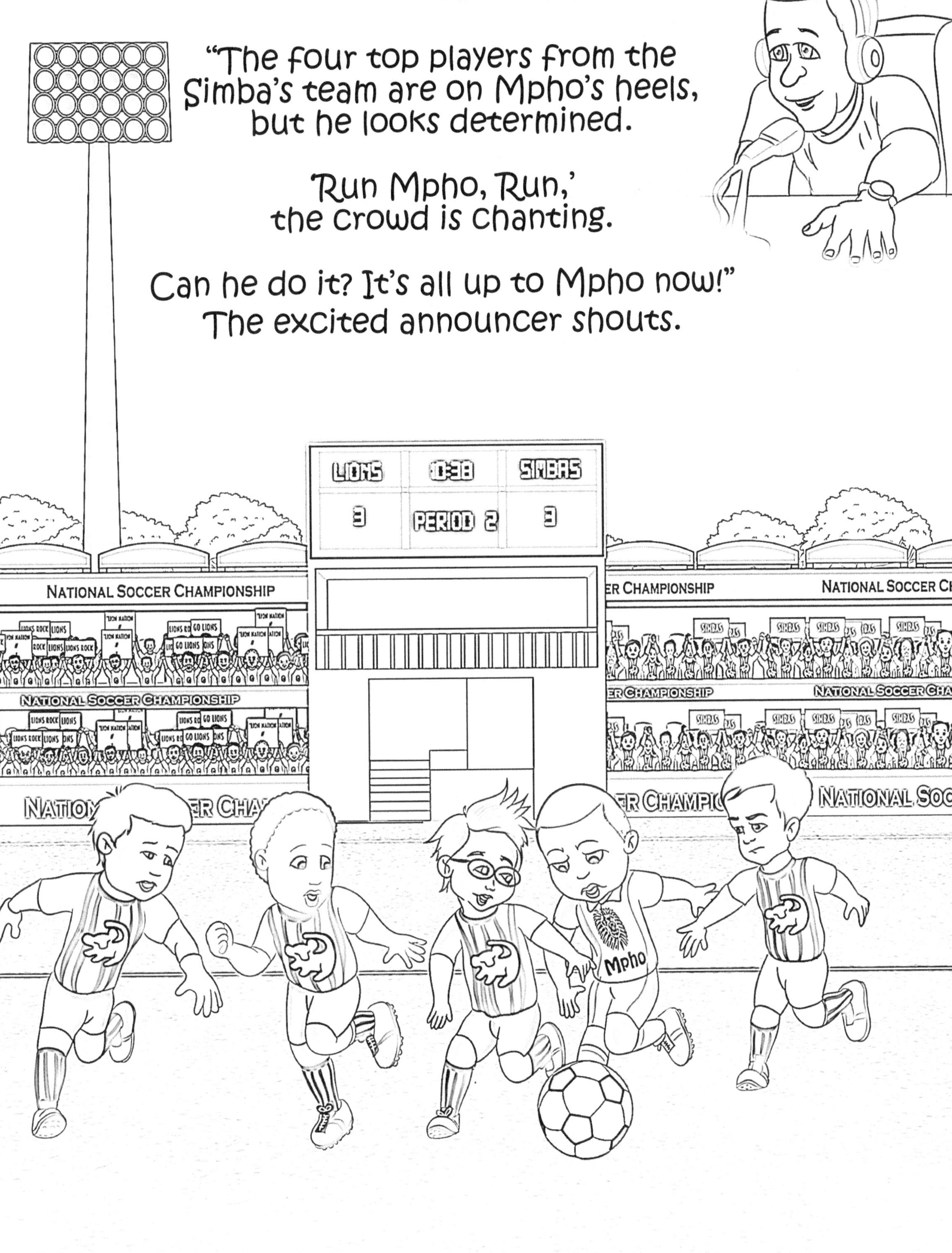

"The four top players from the Simba's team are on Mpho's heels, but he looks determined.

'Run Mpho, Run,' the crowd is chanting.

Can he do it? It's all up to Mpho now!" The excited announcer shouts.

LIONS 0:38 SIMBAS
3 PERIOD 2 3

NATIONAL SOCCER CHAMPIONSHIP

Mpho

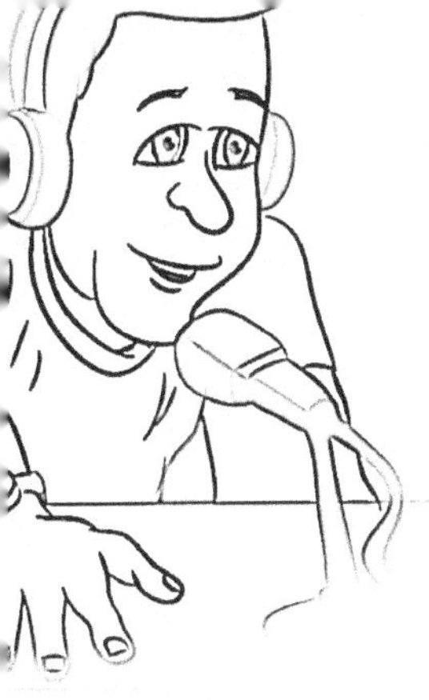

"He draws his foot back as far as he can,
and gives the ball a mighty kick toward the goal.
The ball is in the air with seconds left in the big game.
Can he get it past the Simba goalie?"
The announcer proclaims.

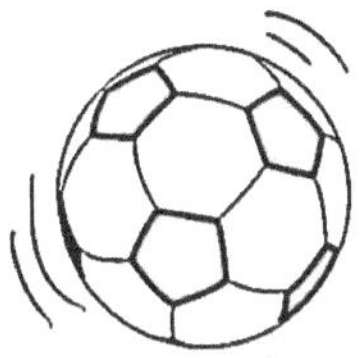

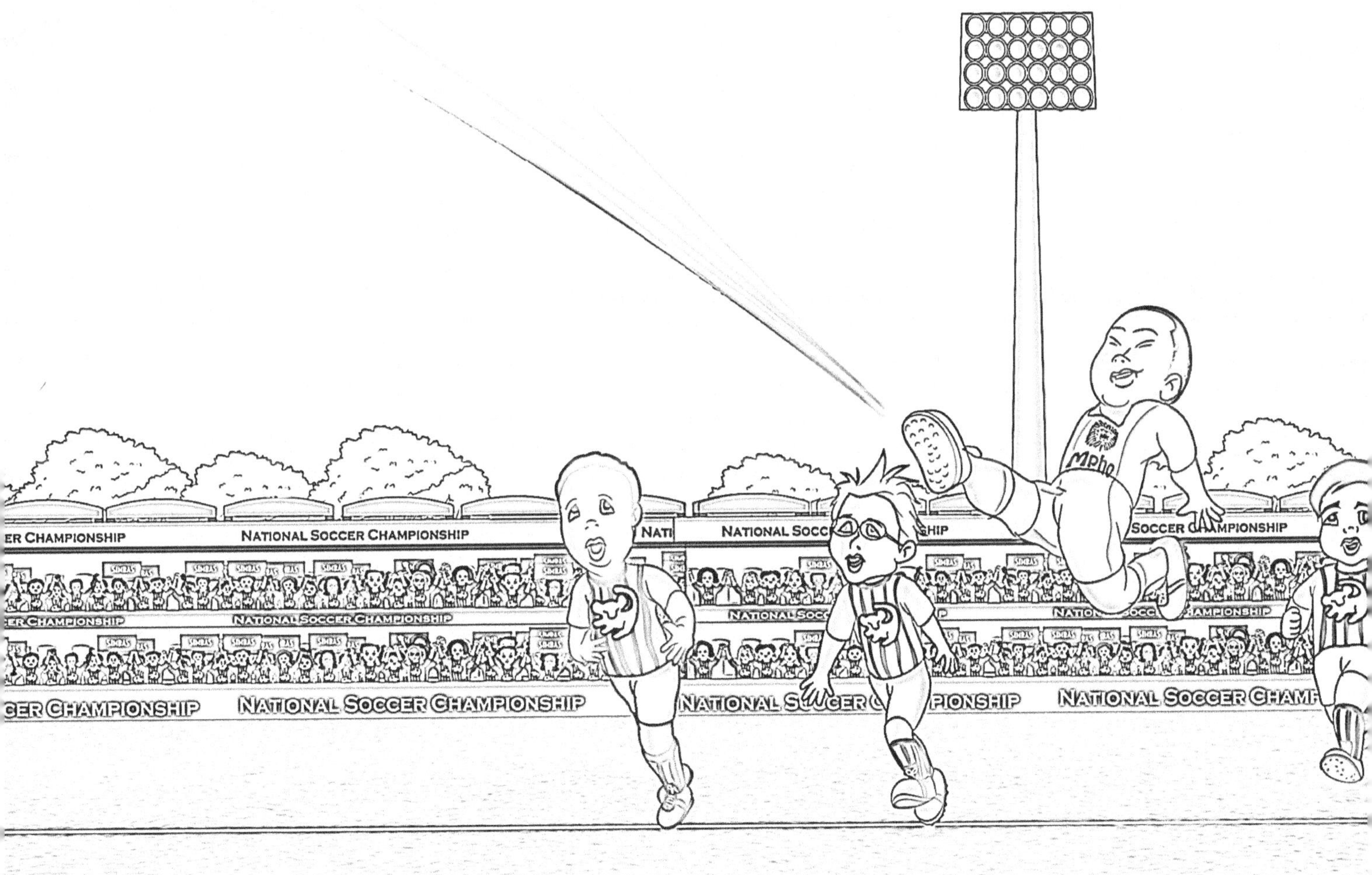

The Simbas goalie dives to block the ball.
Will he stop the Lions from winning
the big championship?

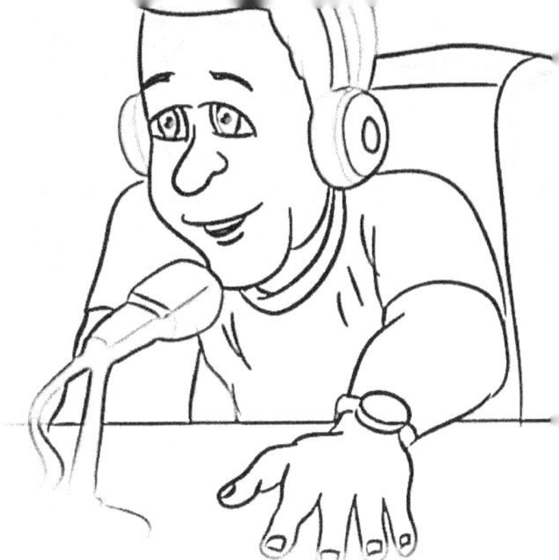

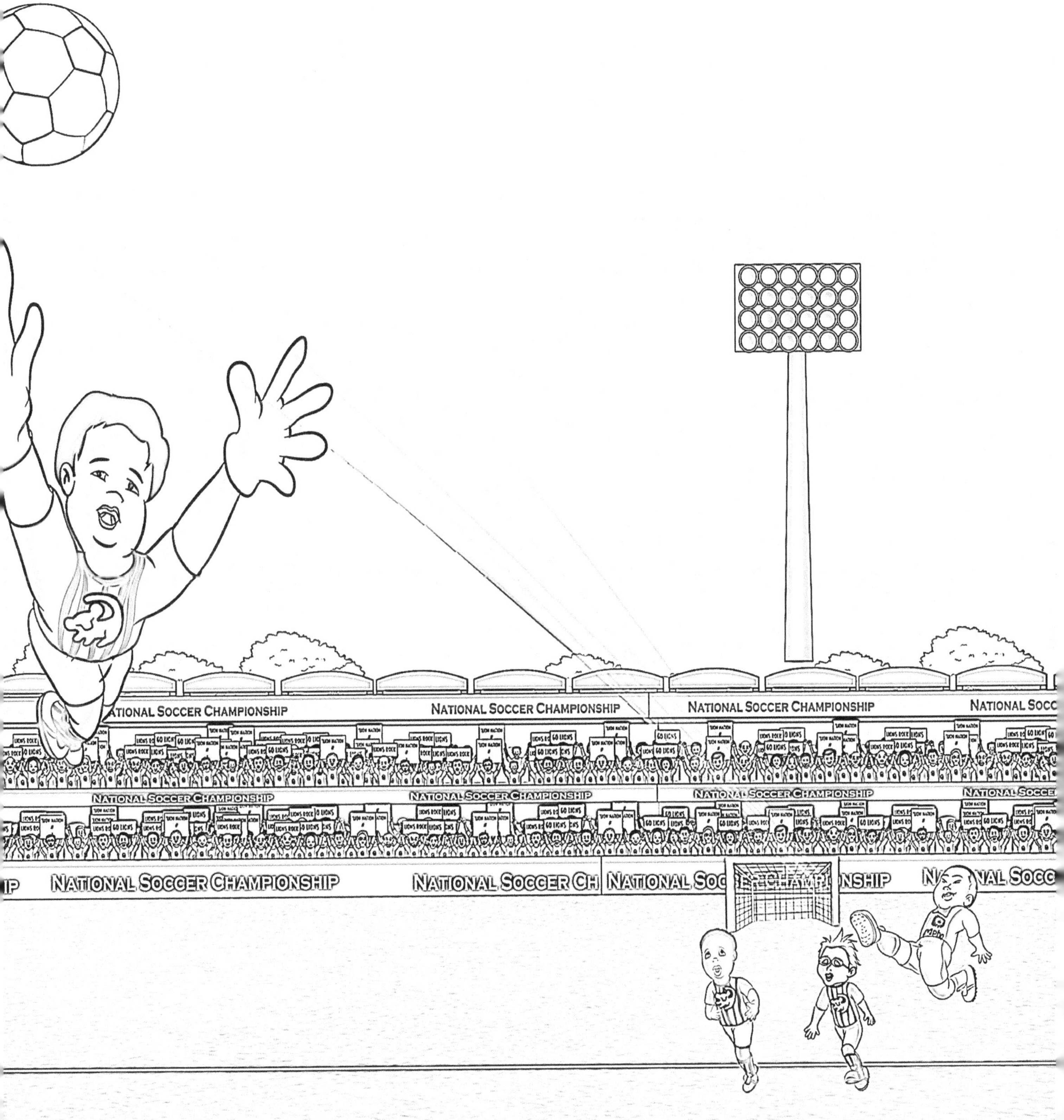

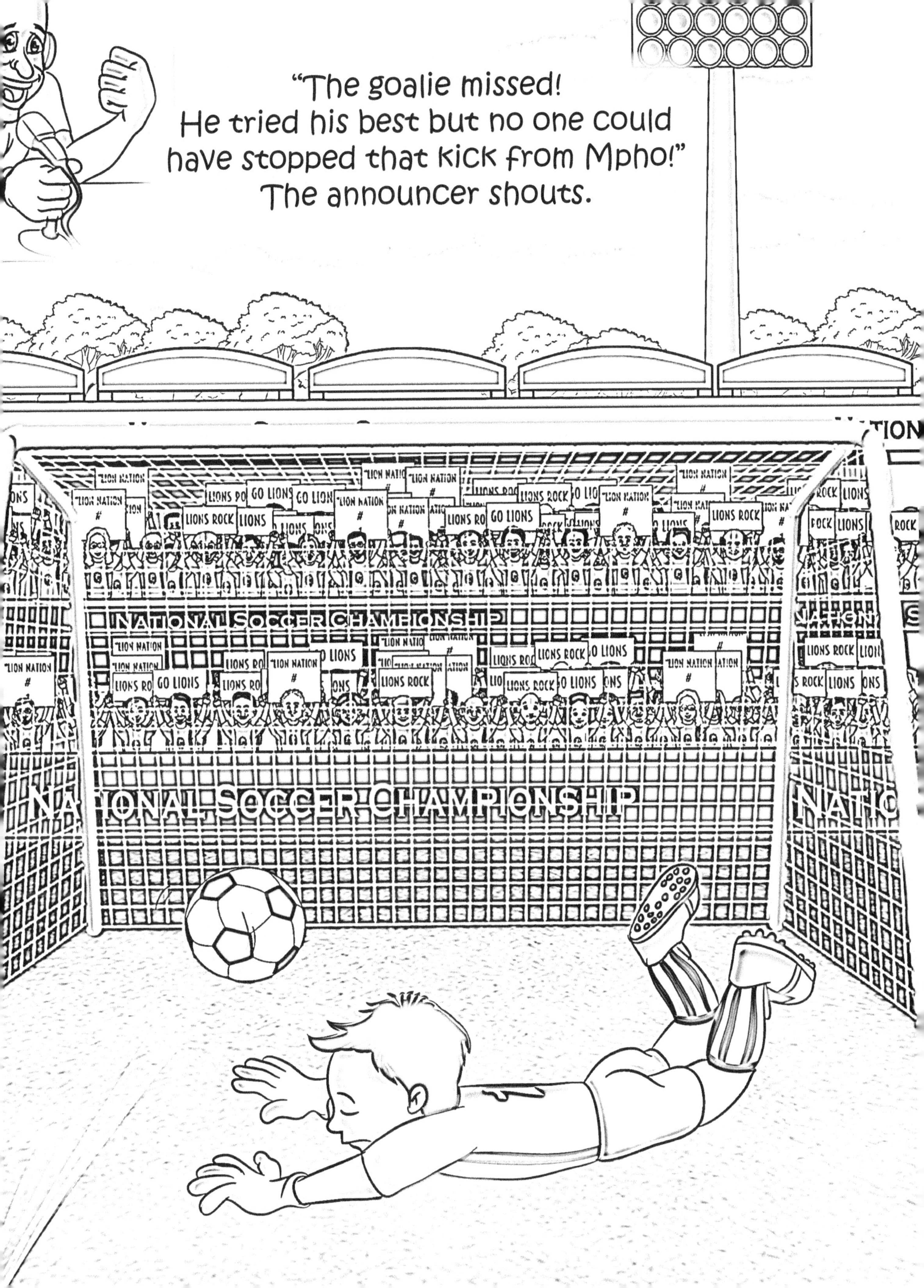

"The goalie missed!
He tried his best but no one could
have stopped that kick from Mpho!"
The announcer shouts.

NATIONAL SOCCER CHAMPIONSHIP

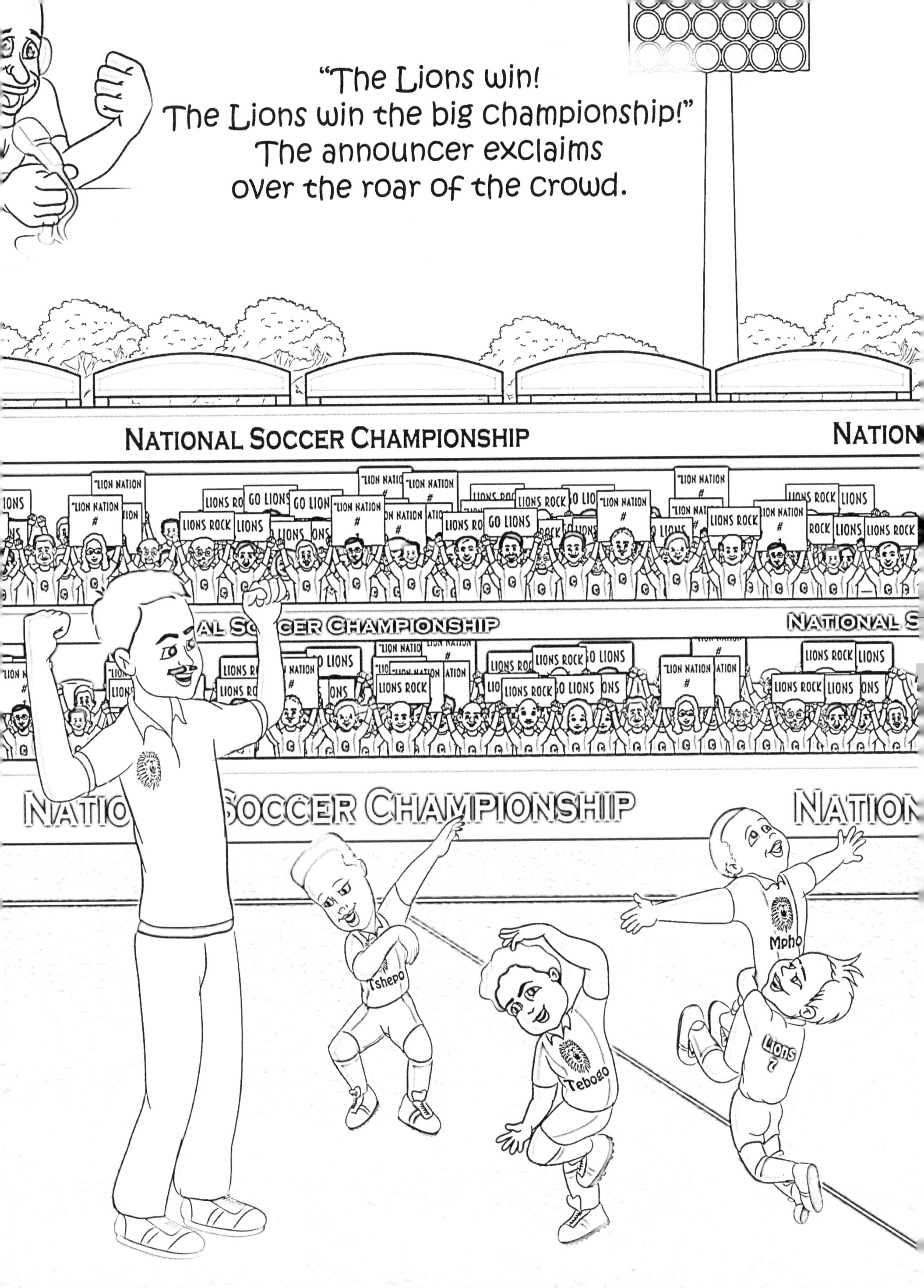

"The Lions win!
The Lions win the big championship!"
The announcer exclaims
over the roar of the crowd.

NATIONAL SOCCER CHAMPIONSHIP
NATION

"LION NATION #
LIONS ROCK
GO LIONS
GO LION
LION NATION
LIONS ROCK LIONS

NATIONAL SOCCER CHAMPIONSHIP
NATIONAL S

NATIO SOCCER CHAMPIONSHIP
NATION

Tshepo
Tebogo
Mpho
Lions 7

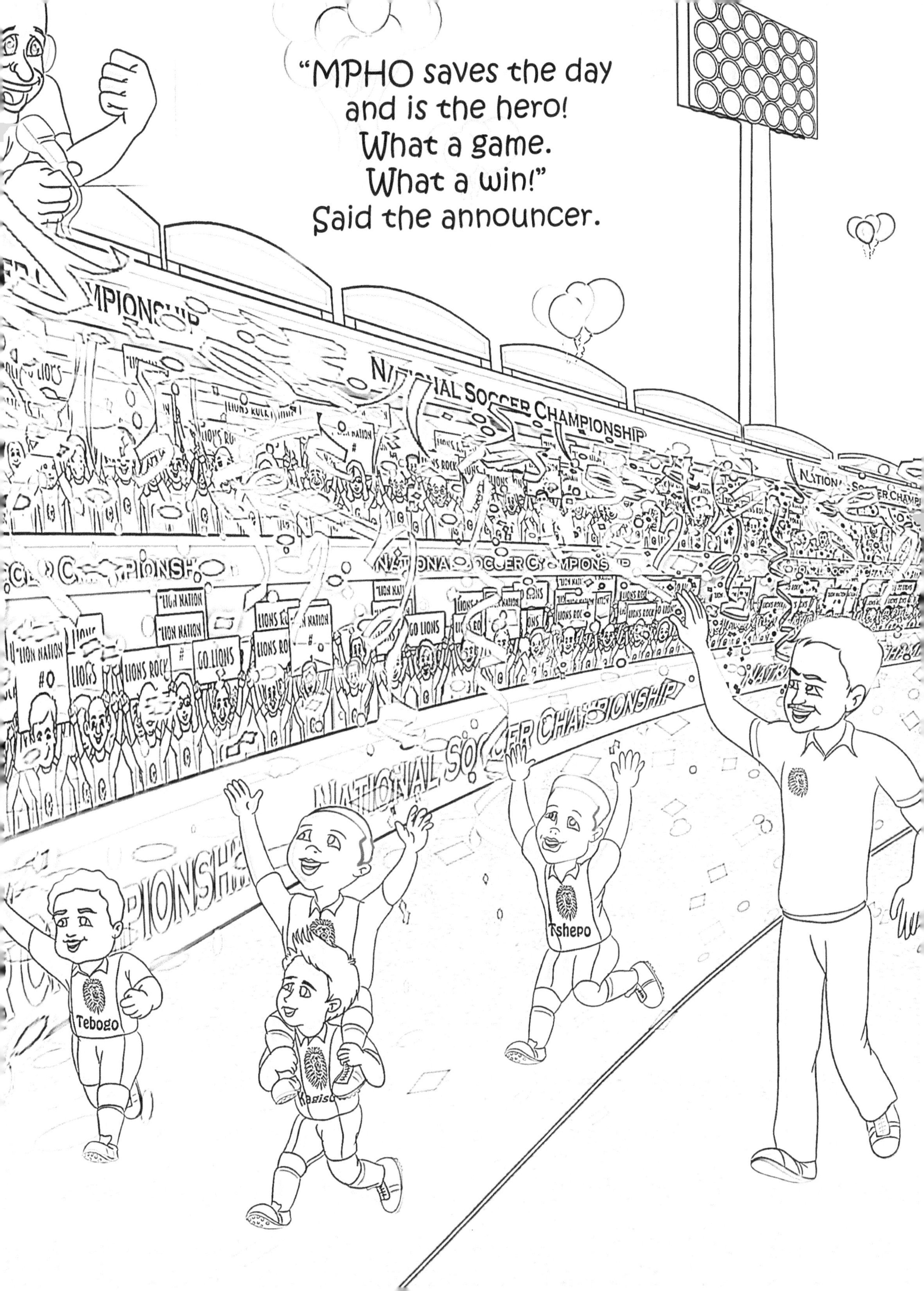

"MPHO saves the day
and is the hero!
What a game.
What a win!"
Said the announcer.

NATIONAL SOCCER CHAMPIONSHIP
Tebogo
Tshepo

"Mpho, I'm so proud of you.
What will you do to celebrate?" The coach asked.

"I think I will invite my teammates
for ice cream." Mpho said.

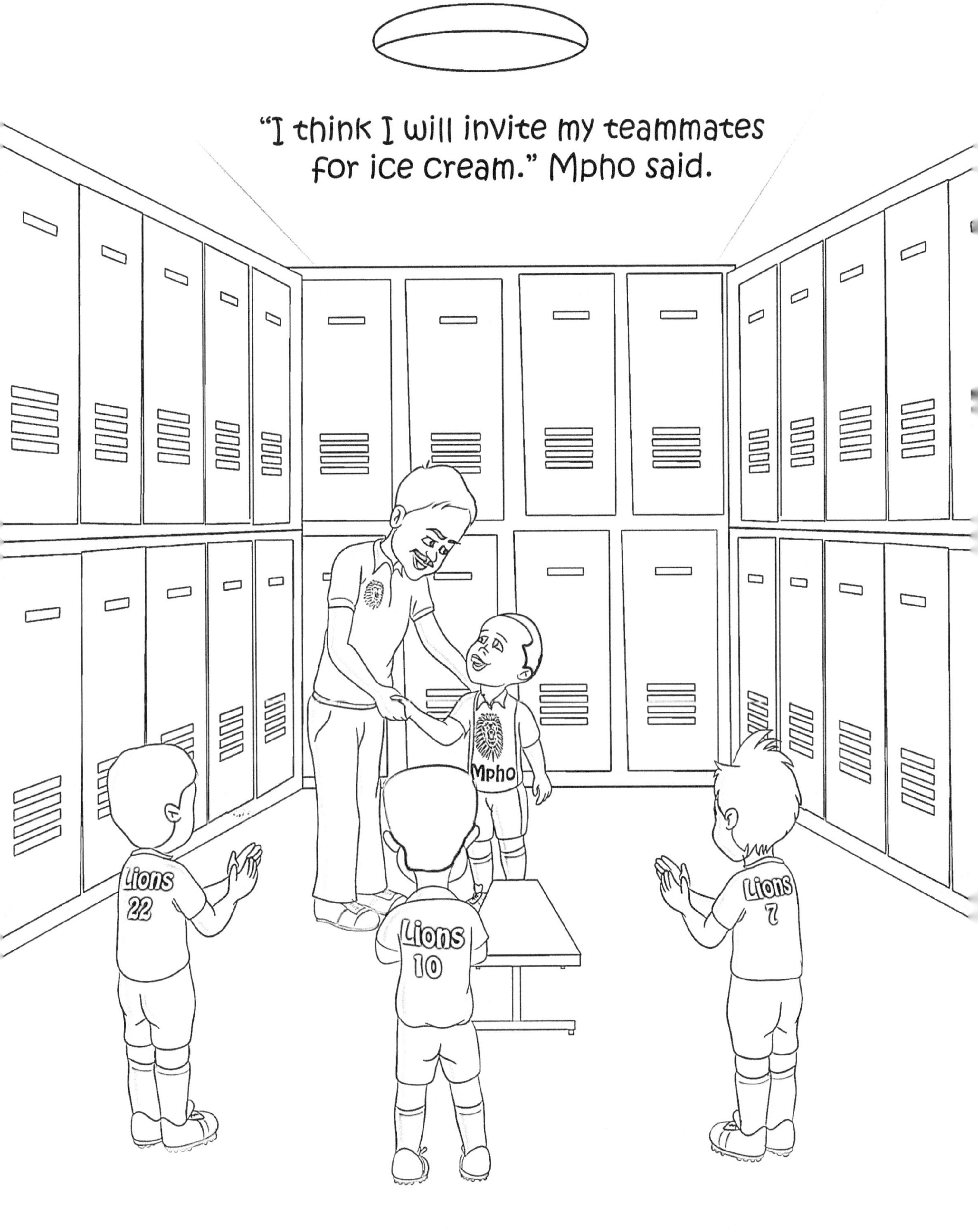

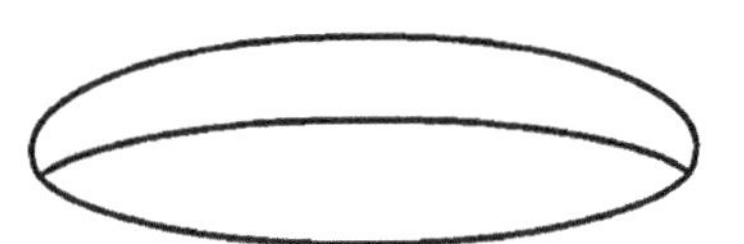

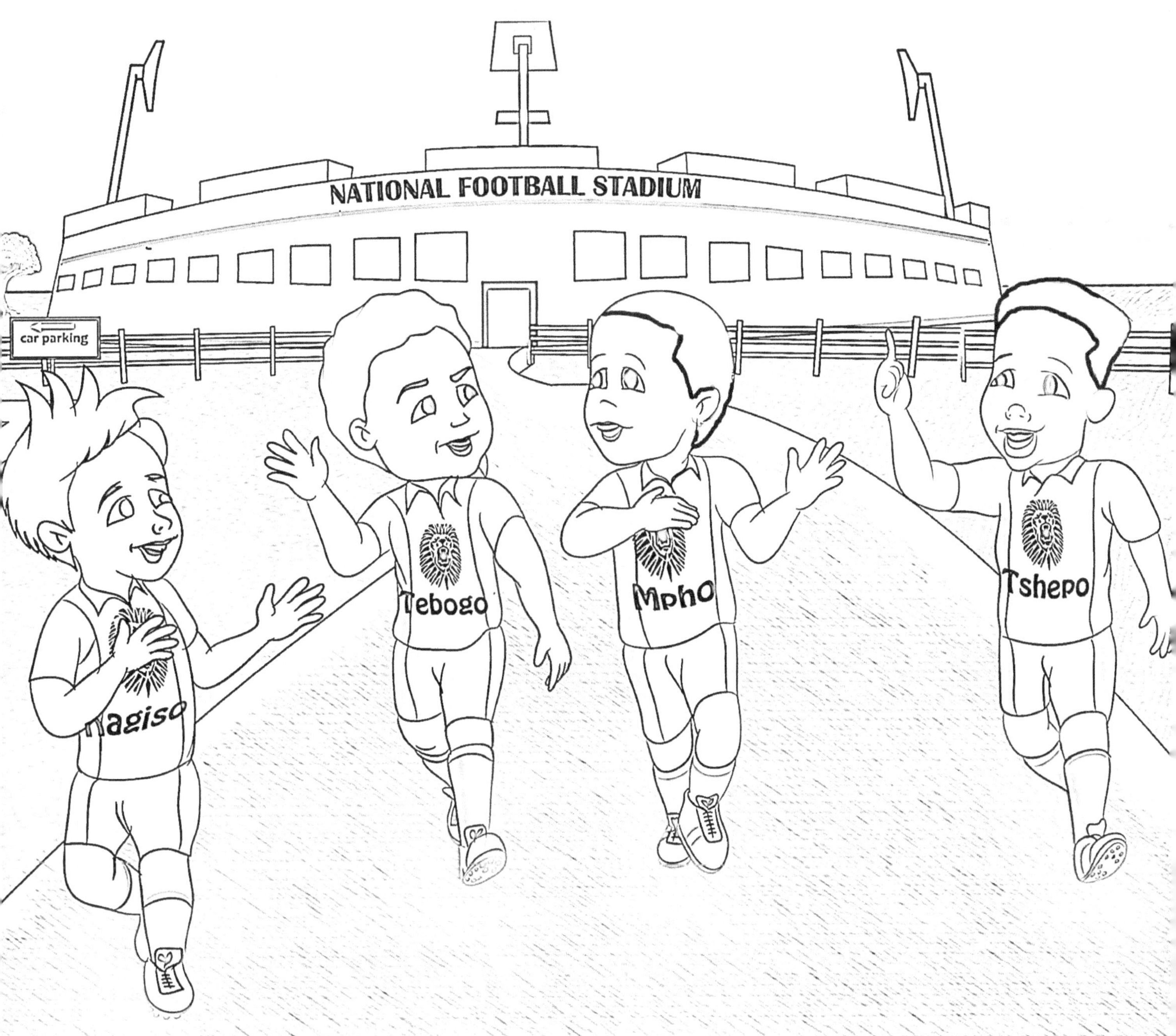

"Wow, this is the best day of my life." Said Tshepo.

"Me too!" Said Kagiso.

"Thanks to Mpho, this is a day
I will never forget!" said Tebogo.

"Thanks," Mpho smiled gratefully.

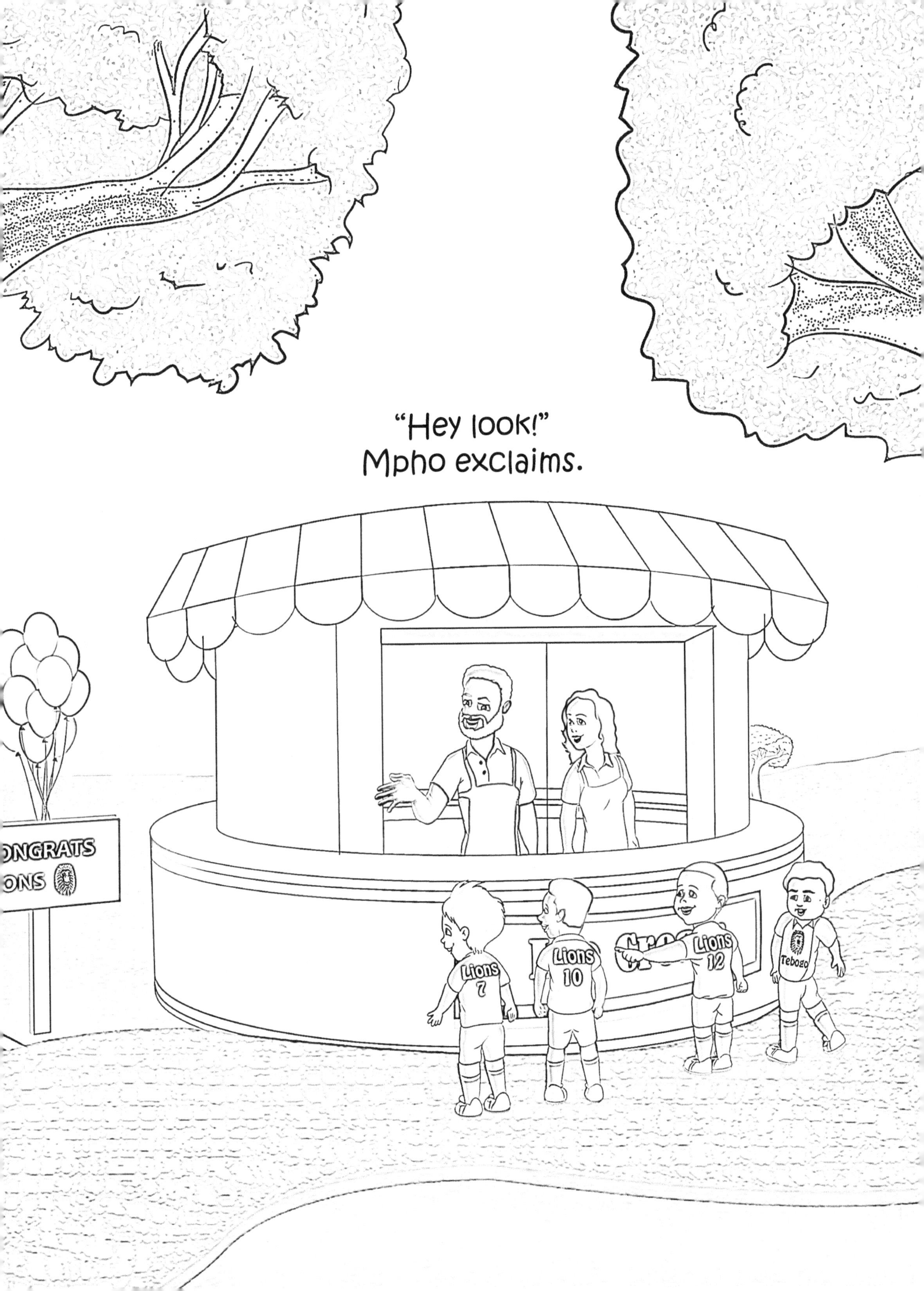

"Hey look!"
Mpho exclaims.

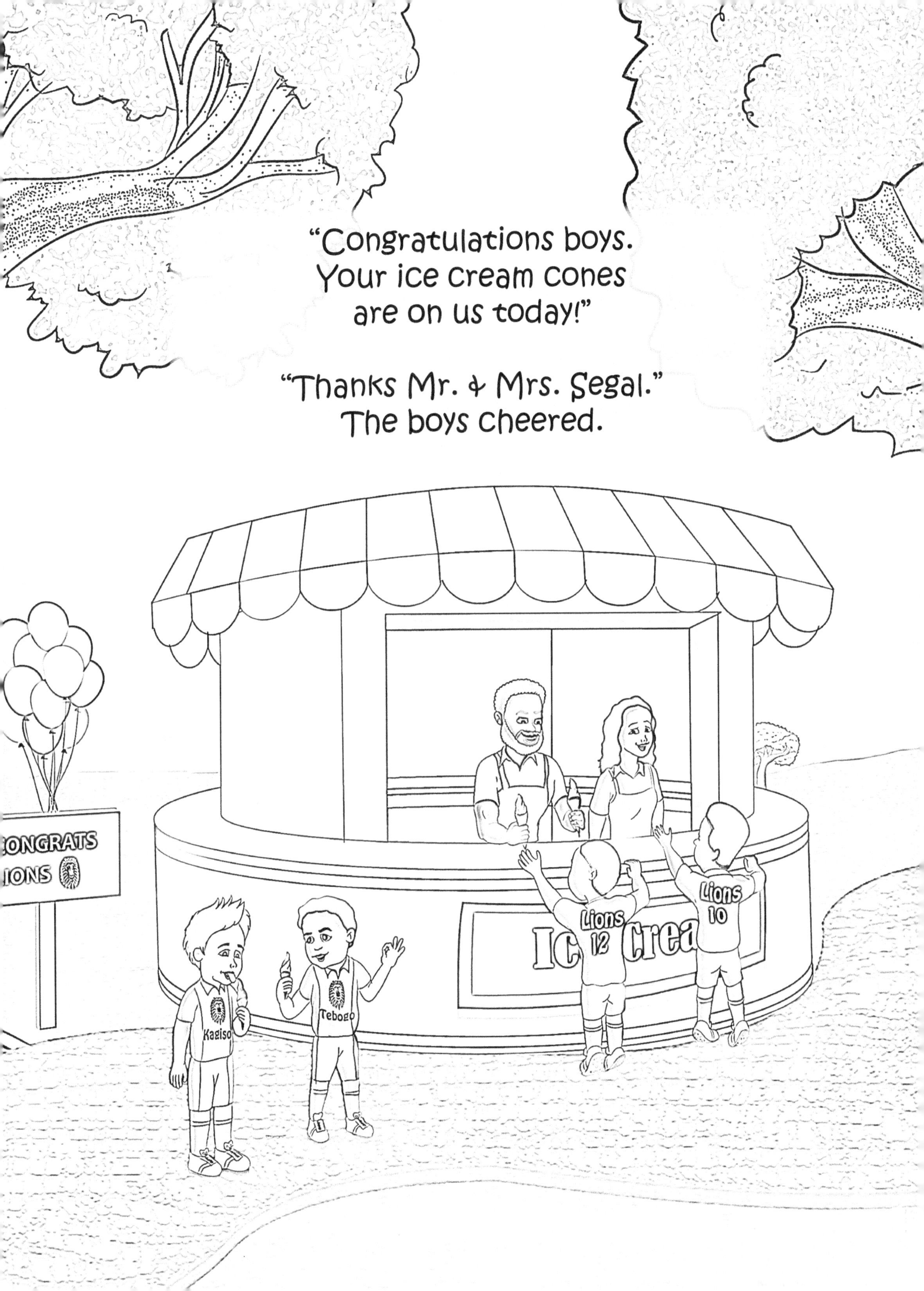

"Congratulations boys.
Your ice cream cones
are on us today!"

"Thanks Mr. & Mrs. Segal."
The boys cheered.

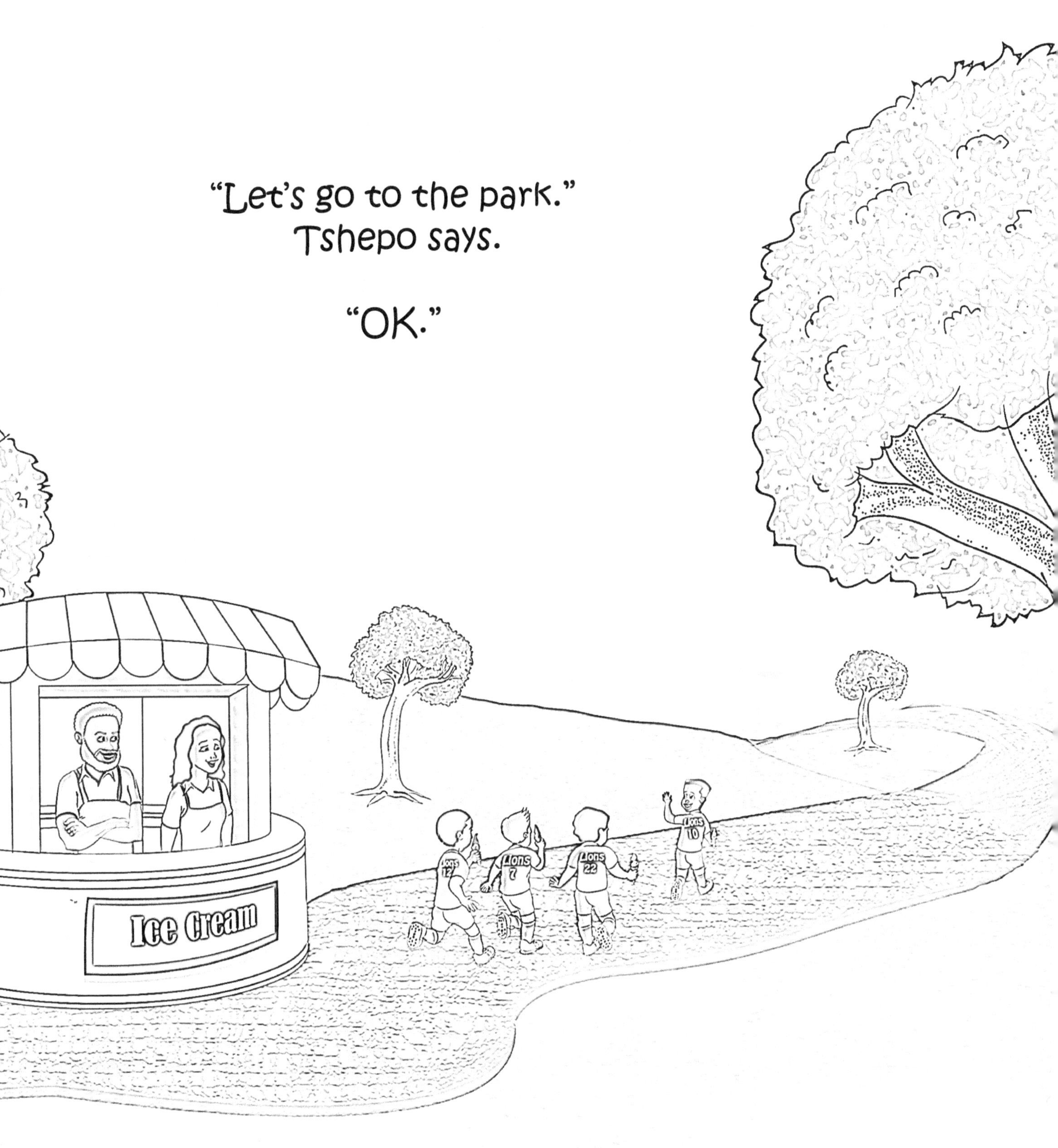

"Let's go to the park."
Tshepo says.

"OK."

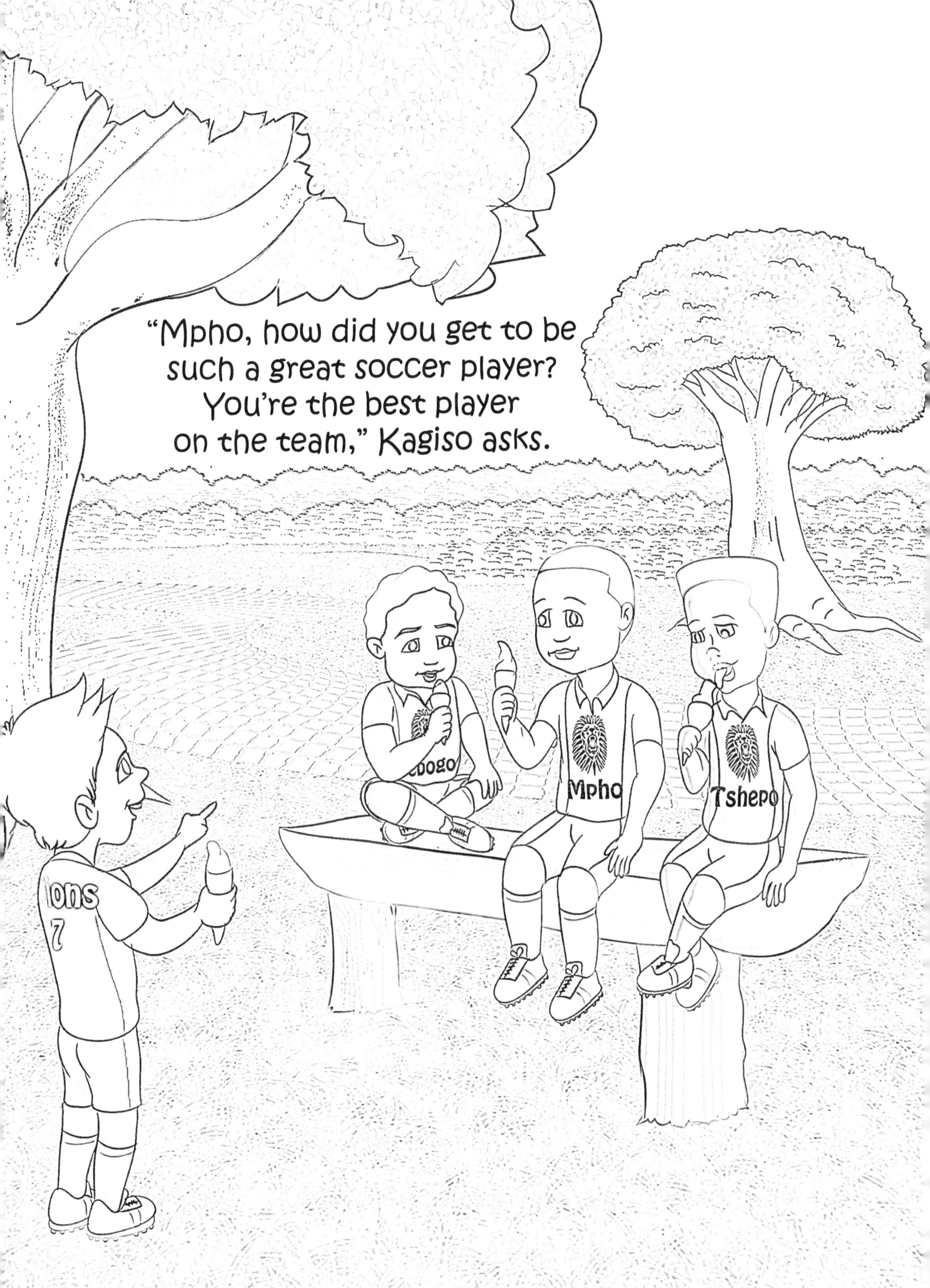

"Mpho, how did you get to be such a great soccer player? You're the best player on the team," Kagiso asks.
Odogo
Mpho
Tshepo
ions
7

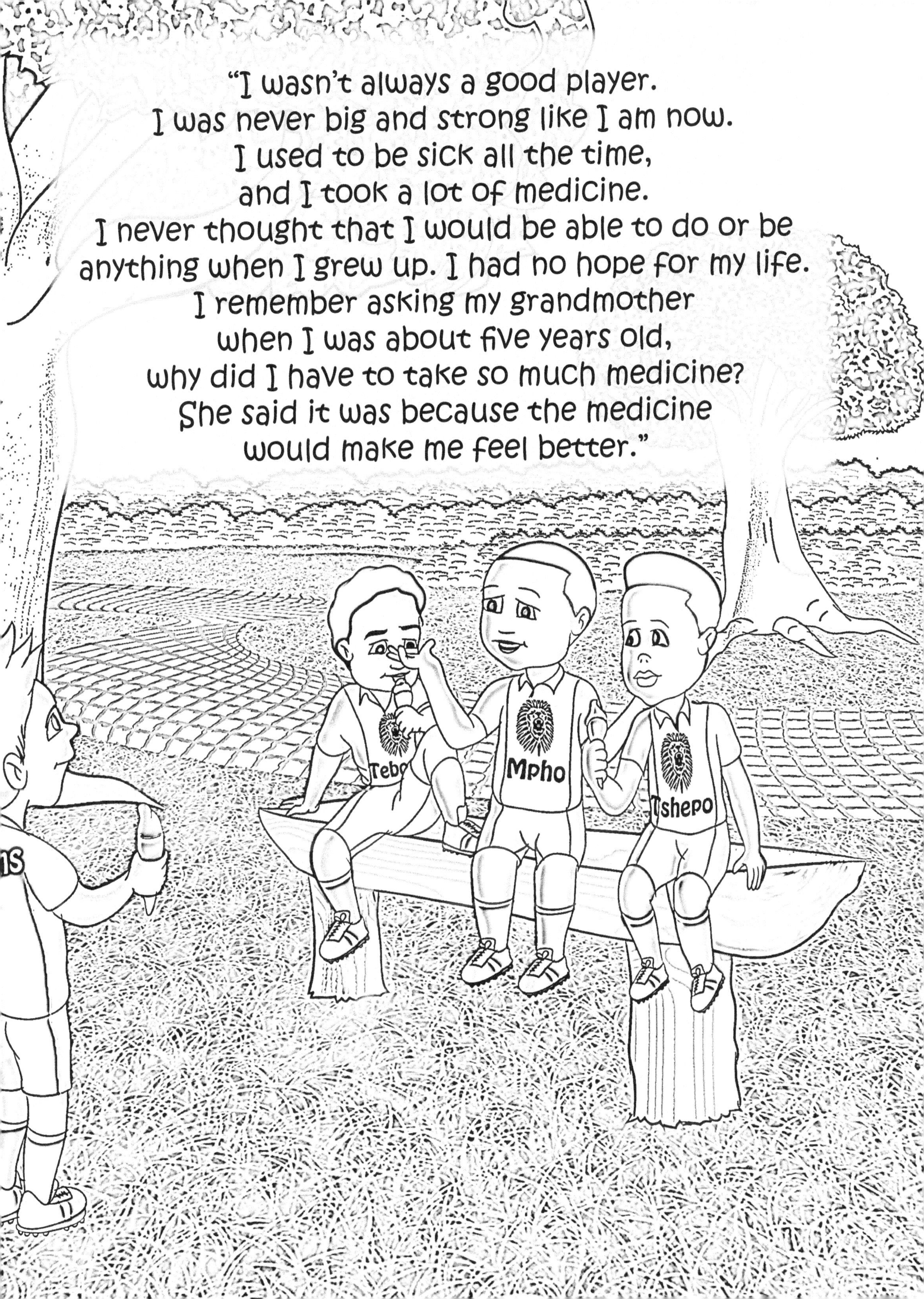

"I wasn't always a good player.
I was never big and strong like I am now.
I used to be sick all the time,
and I took a lot of medicine.
I never thought that I would be able to do or be
anything when I grew up. I had no hope for my life.
I remember asking my grandmother
when I was about five years old,
why did I have to take so much medicine?
She said it was because the medicine
would make me feel better."
Tebo
Mpho
Tshepo

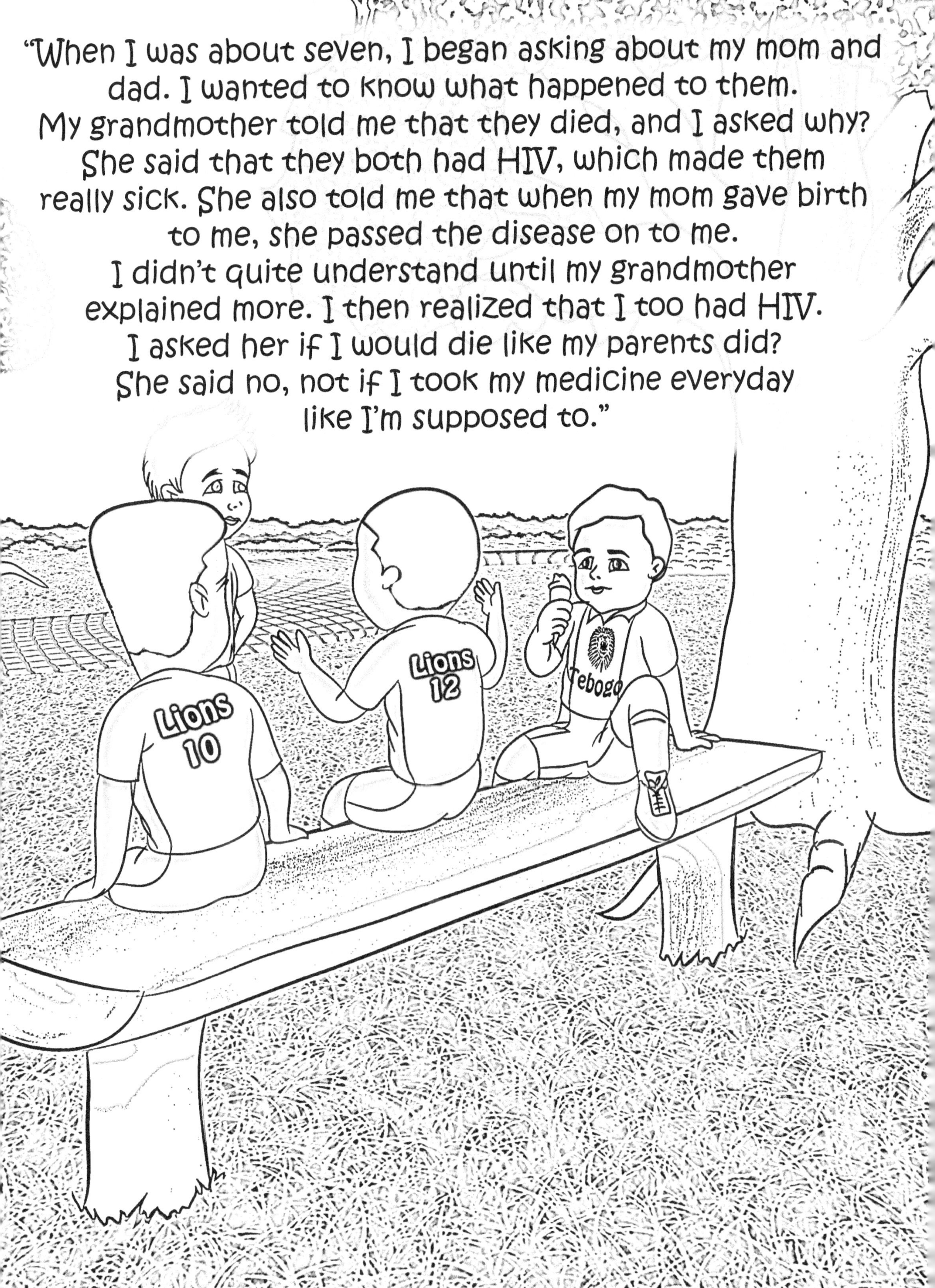

"When I was about seven, I began asking about my mom and dad. I wanted to know what happened to them. My grandmother told me that they died, and I asked why? She said that they both had HIV, which made them really sick. She also told me that when my mom gave birth to me, she passed the disease on to me. I didn't quite understand until my grandmother explained more. I then realized that I too had HIV. I asked her if I would die like my parents did? She said no, not if I took my medicine everyday like I'm supposed to."
Lions 10
Lions 12
Tebogo

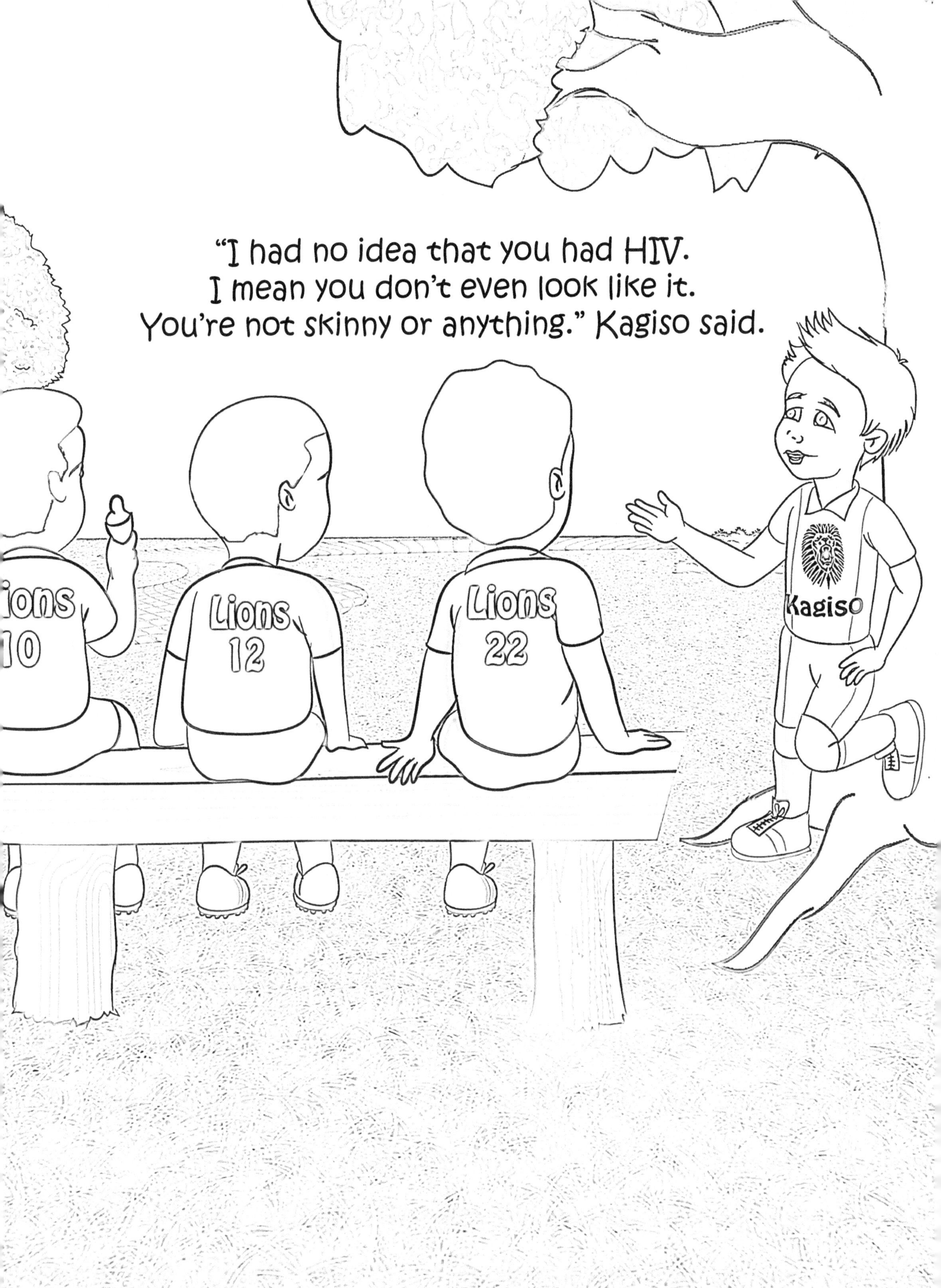

"I had no idea that you had HIV.
I mean you don't even look like it.
You're not skinny or anything." Kagiso said.
Lions
10
Lions
12
Lions
22
Kagiso

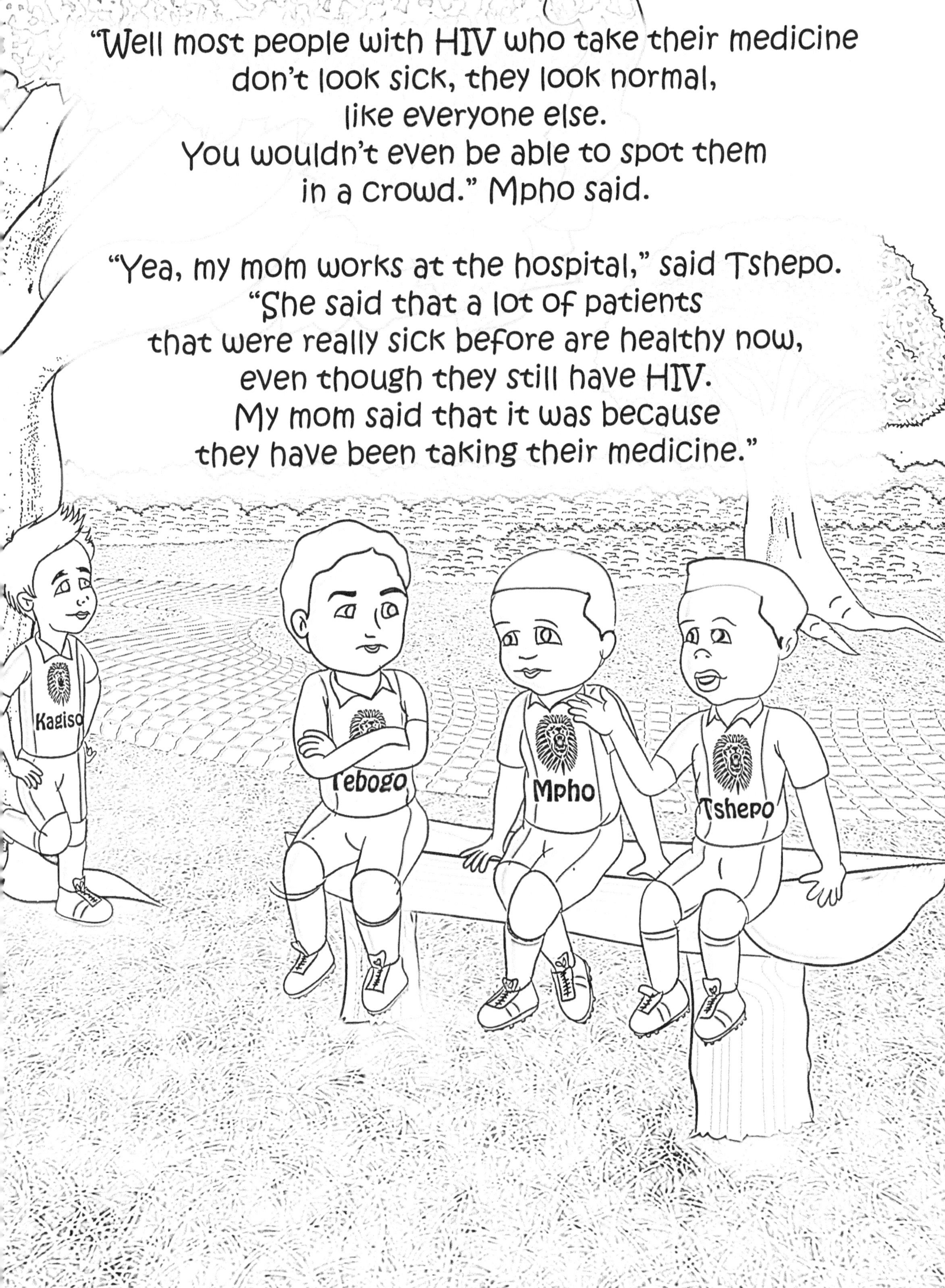

"Well most people with HIV who take their medicine
don't look sick, they look normal,
like everyone else.
You wouldn't even be able to spot them
in a crowd." Mpho said.

"Yea, my mom works at the hospital," said Tshepo.
"She said that a lot of patients
that were really sick before are healthy now,
even though they still have HIV.
My mom said that it was because
they have been taking their medicine."

Kagiso
Tebogo
Mpho
Tshepo

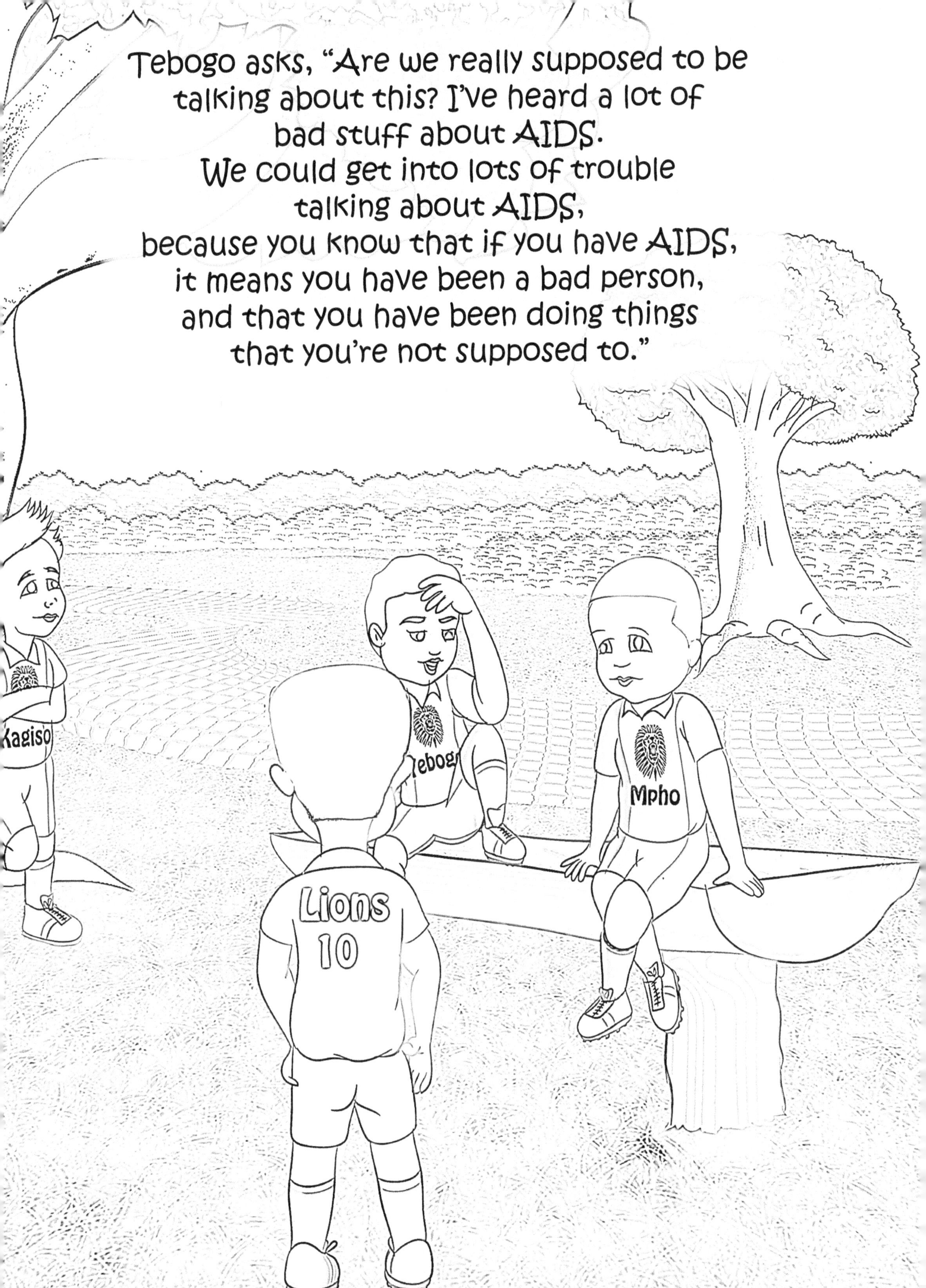

Tebogo asks, "Are we really supposed to be talking about this? I've heard a lot of bad stuff about AIDS.
We could get into lots of trouble talking about AIDS,
because you know that if you have AIDS, it means you have been a bad person, and that you have been doing things that you're not supposed to."
Kagiso
Tebogo
Mpho
Lions
10

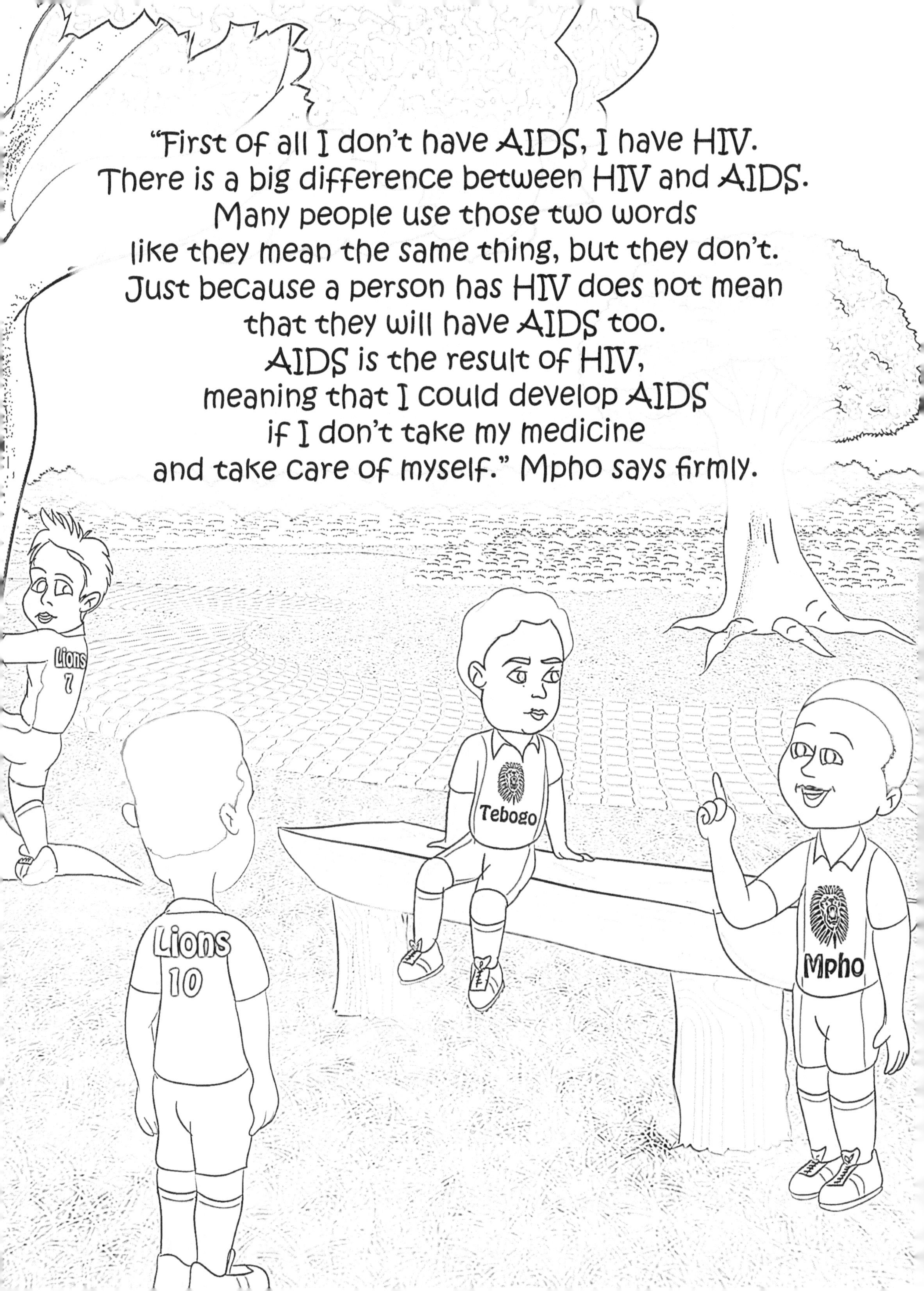

"First of all I don't have AIDS, I have HIV.
There is a big difference between HIV and AIDS.
Many people use those two words
like they mean the same thing, but they don't.
Just because a person has HIV does not mean
that they will have AIDS too.
AIDS is the result of HIV,
meaning that I could develop AIDS
if I don't take my medicine
and take care of myself." Mpho says firmly.
Lions
7
Lions
10
Tebogo
Mpho

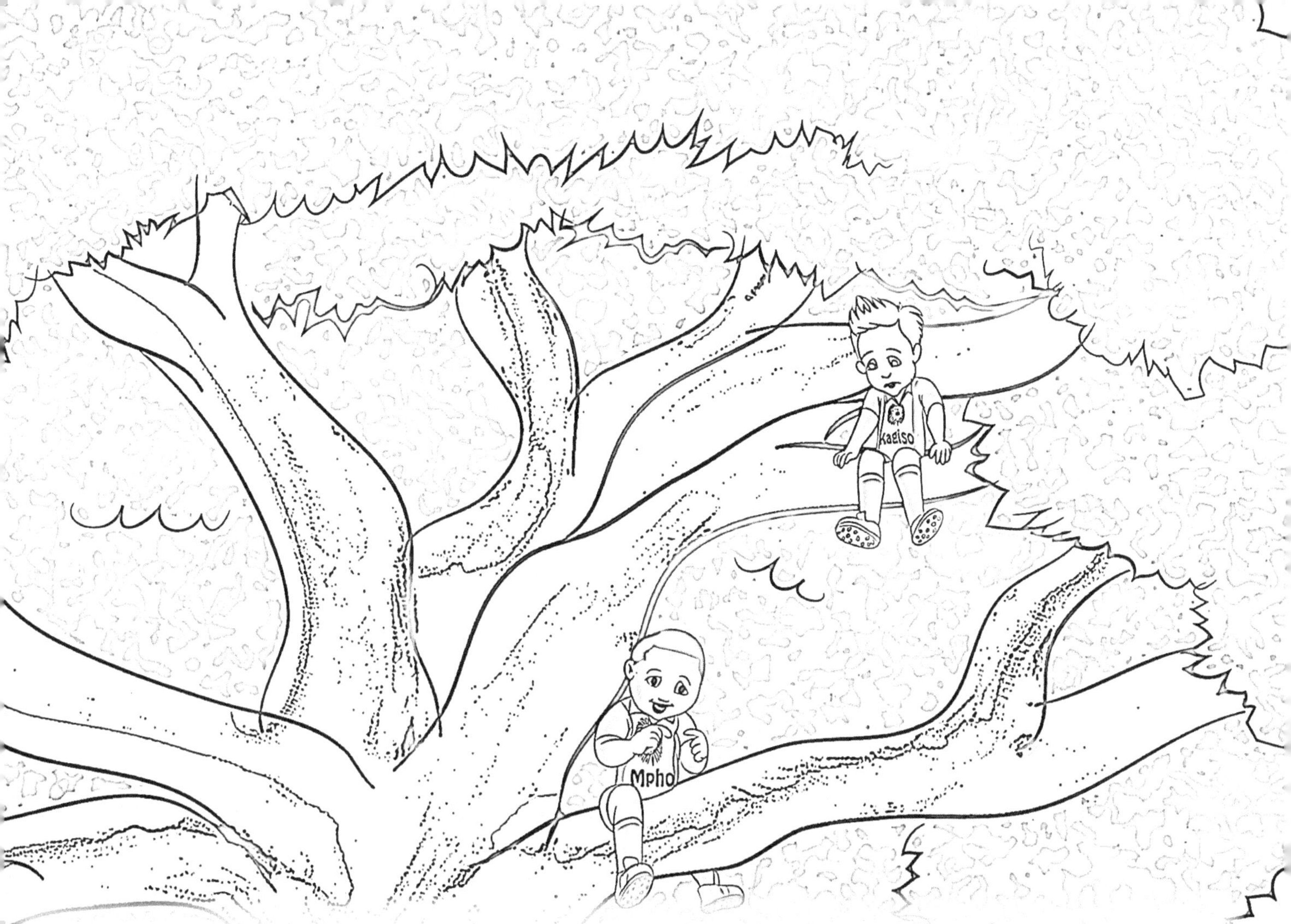

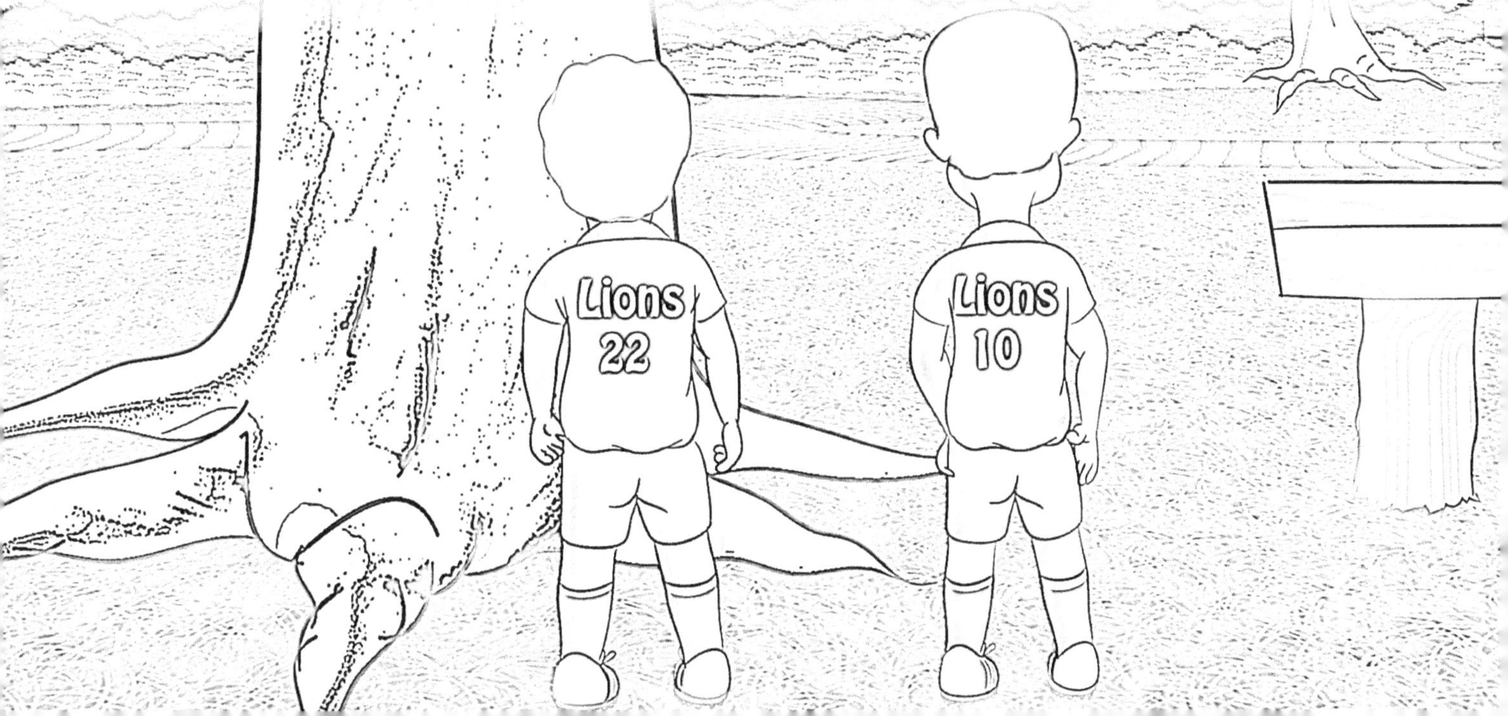

"Having HIV or AIDS doesn't make you a bad person, and it doesn't mean that you've done something bad to get it. Look at me, I was just born, and I got it. Being born is a good thing; you were born too, or else you wouldn't be here today and we wouldn't have won the championship!"

"Oh, I get it. HIV/AIDS are like having a bad cold or the flu. Having it doesn't make you a bad person. It's just an illness!" Tebogo shouts.

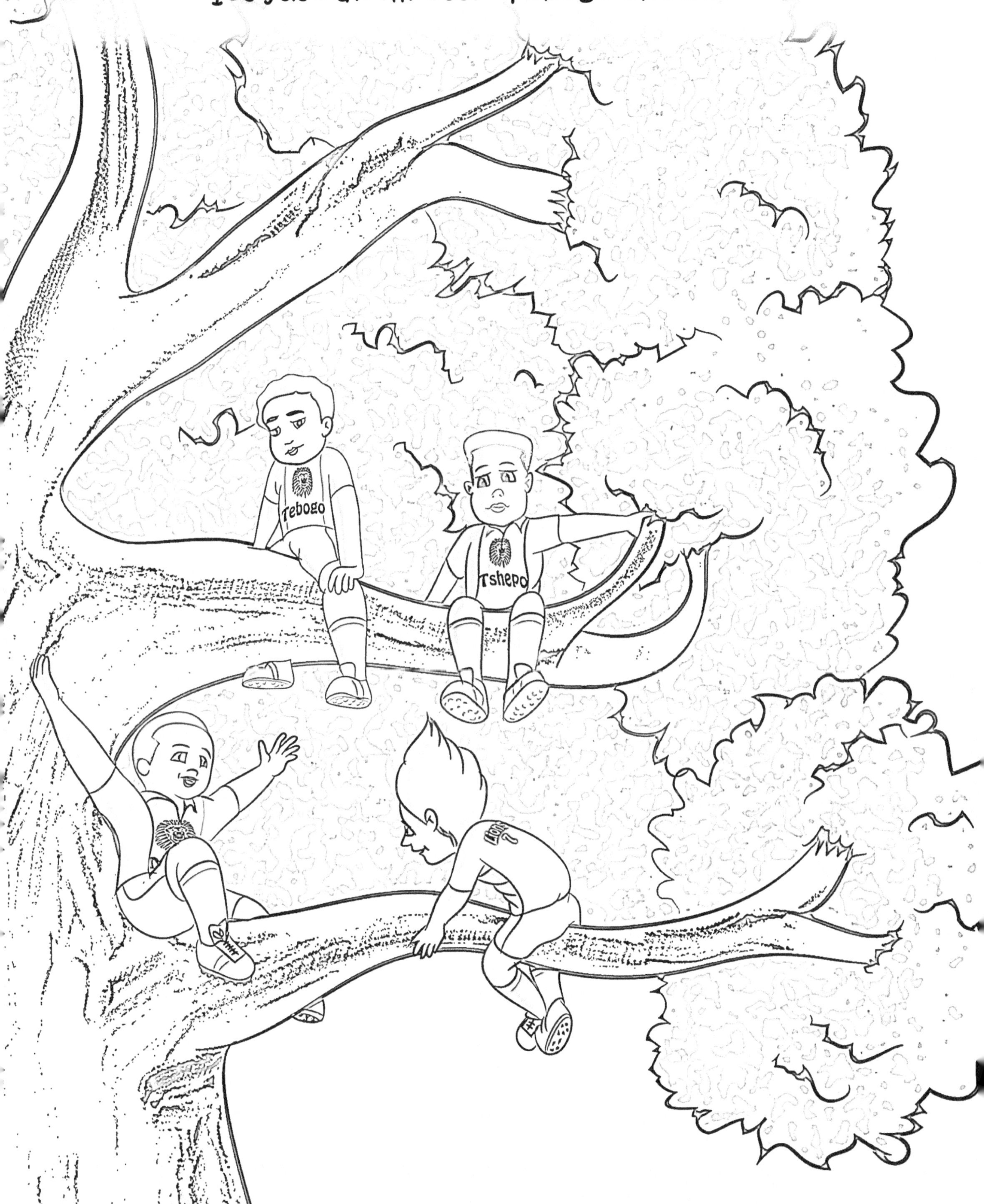

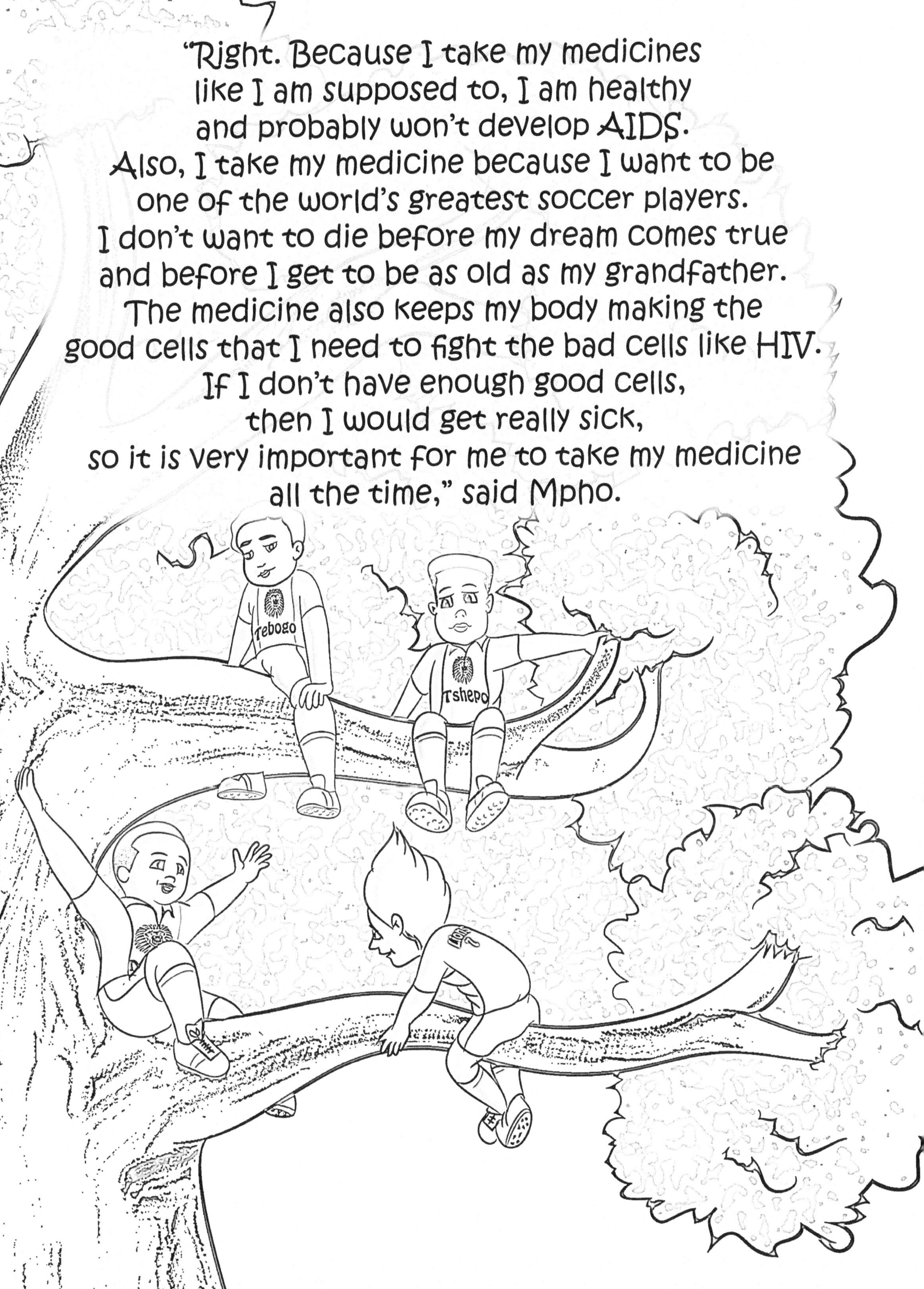

"Right. Because I take my medicines
like I am supposed to, I am healthy
and probably won't develop AIDS.
Also, I take my medicine because I want to be
one of the world's greatest soccer players.
I don't want to die before my dream comes true
and before I get to be as old as my grandfather.
The medicine also keeps my body making the
good cells that I need to fight the bad cells like HIV.
If I don't have enough good cells,
then I would get really sick,
so it is very important for me to take my medicine
all the time," said Mpho.

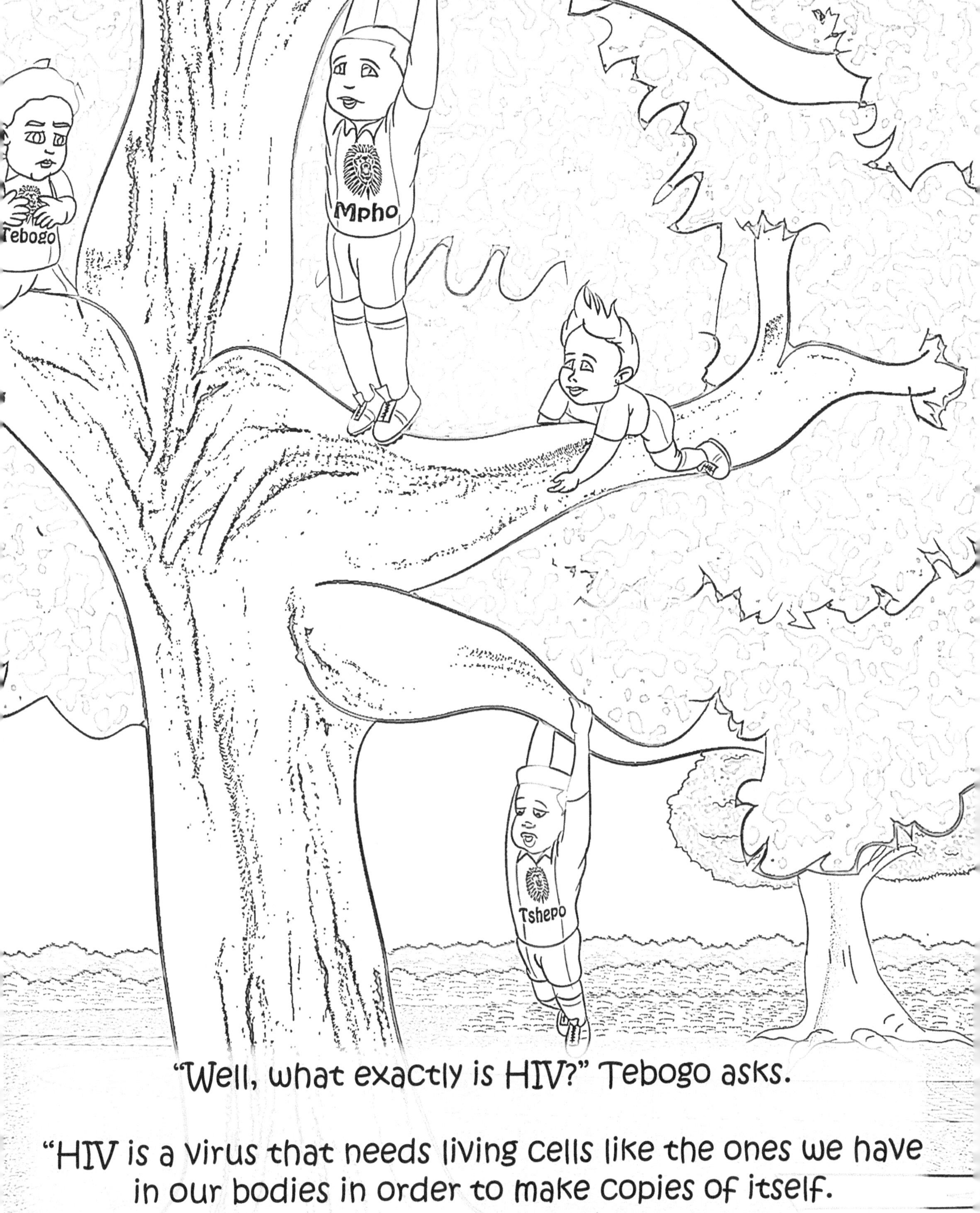

"Well, what exactly is HIV?" Tebogo asks.

"HIV is a virus that needs living cells like the ones we have
in our bodies in order to make copies of itself.
With its new copies HIV infects us,
and kills the good cells that keeps us healthy."
Mpho answers.

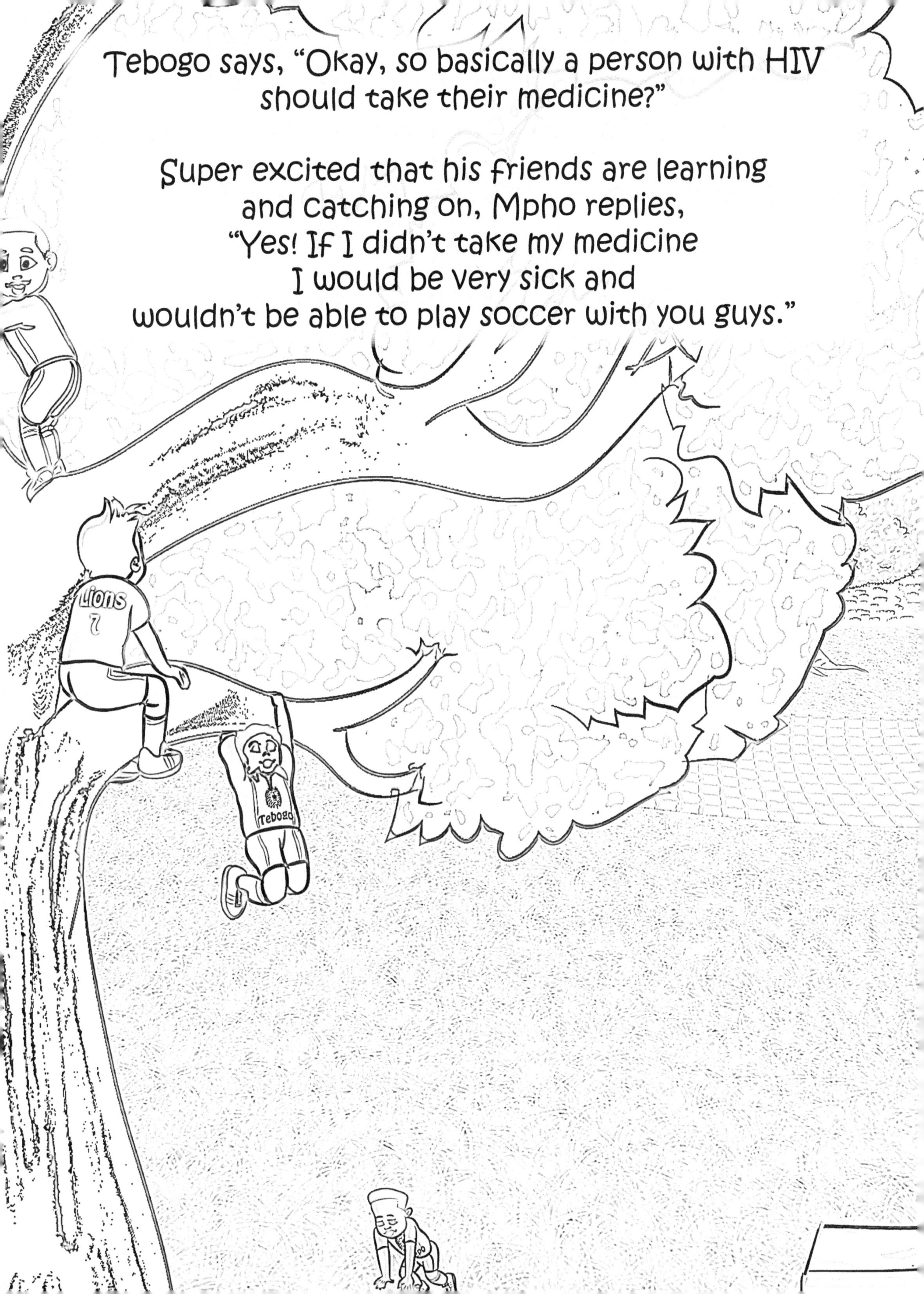

Tebogo says, "Okay, so basically a person with HIV should take their medicine?"

Super excited that his friends are learning and catching on, Mpho replies,
"Yes! If I didn't take my medicine I would be very sick and wouldn't be able to play soccer with you guys."

"You know if my mom knew that you had HIV,
she would probably not let me play with you
or even talk to you." Kagiso said.

"A lot of people feel that way. They think that if they
touch me they will get HIV. That's not true. You cannot
get HIV from sharing a room, or a house, or a fork,
or some food with someone. You can't even get it
from talking to someone with it,
or from sitting by someone with it." Mpho said.

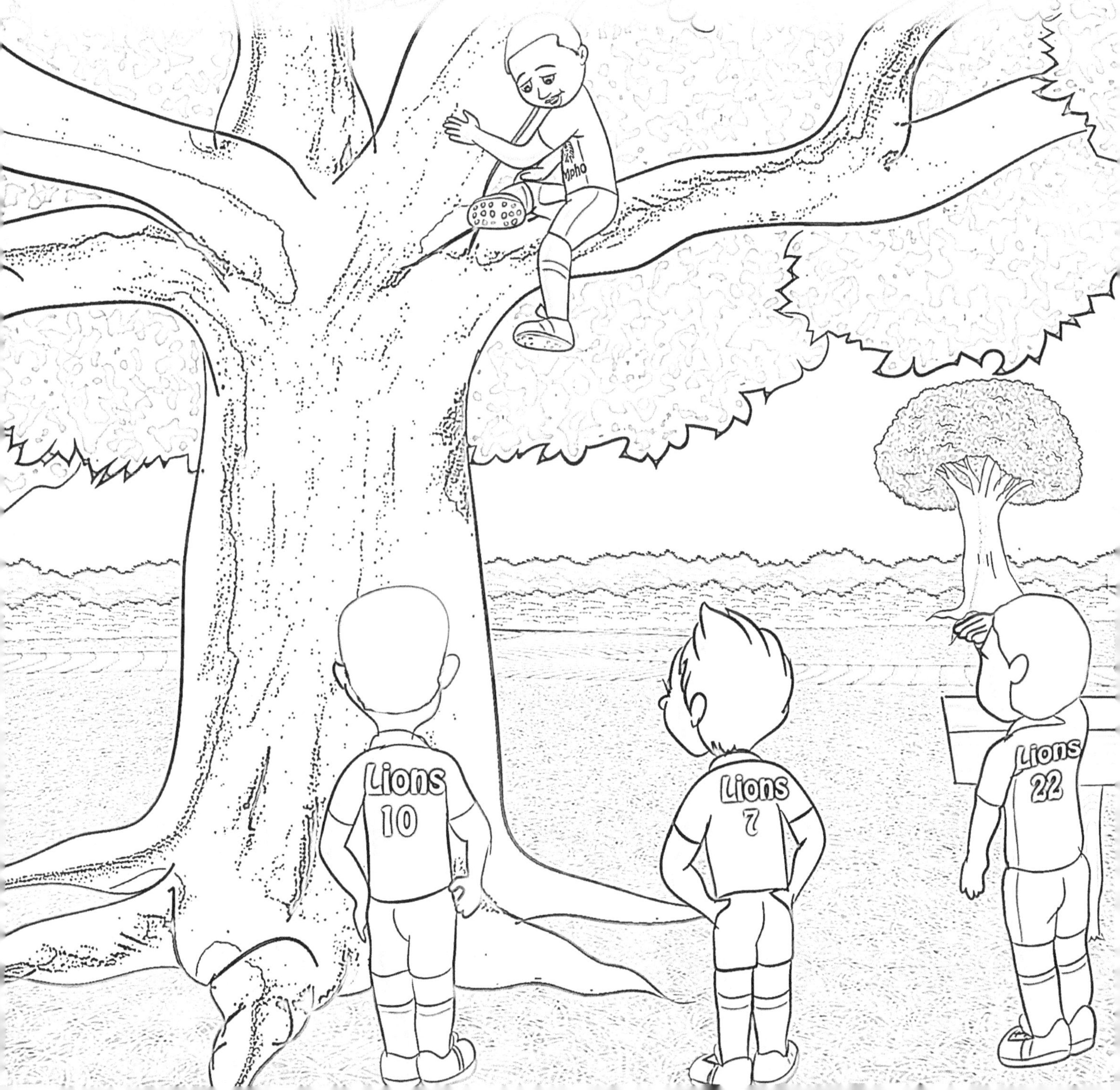

WOW, the boys exclaimed.
"I never knew
it was that hard to get HIV."

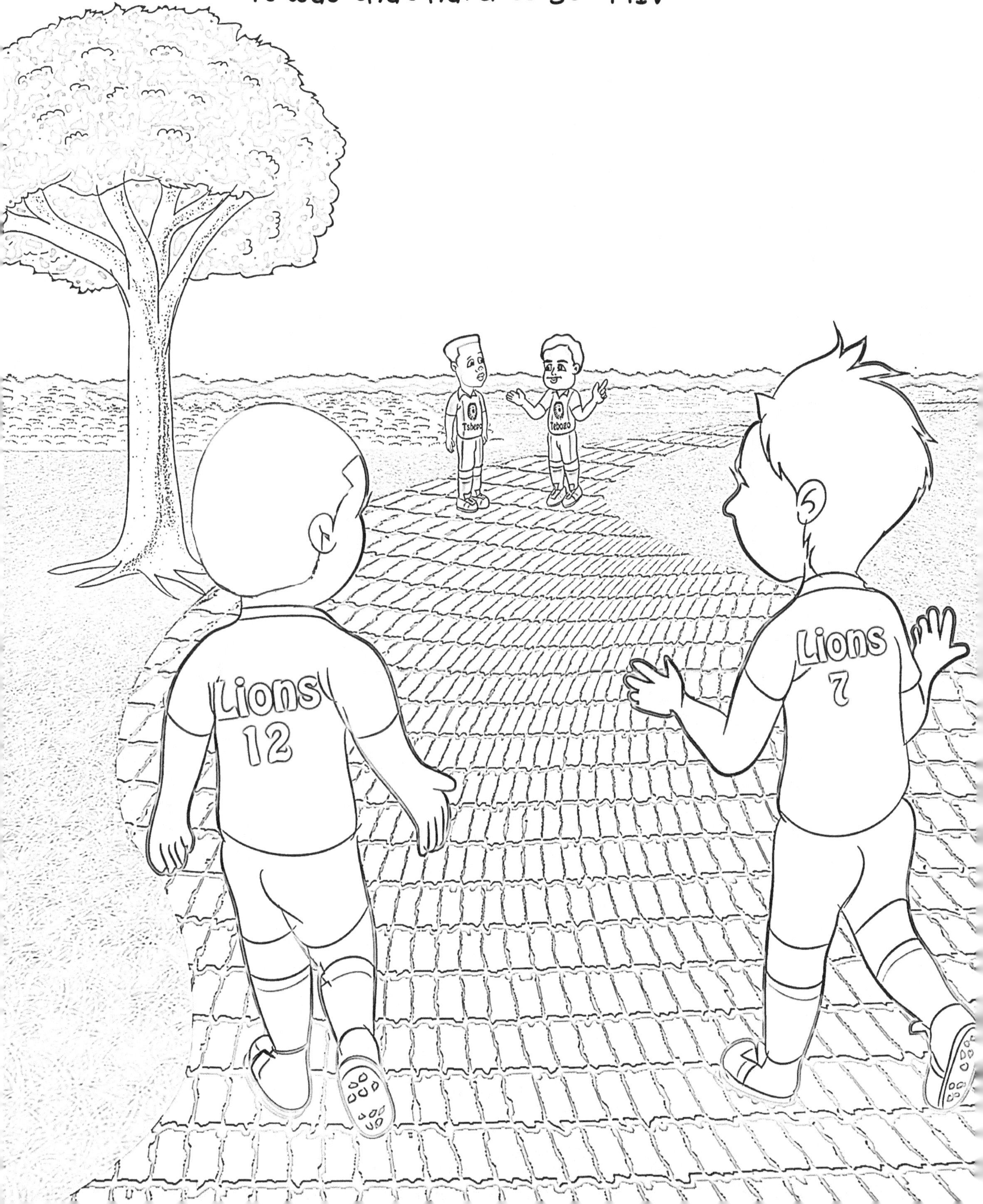

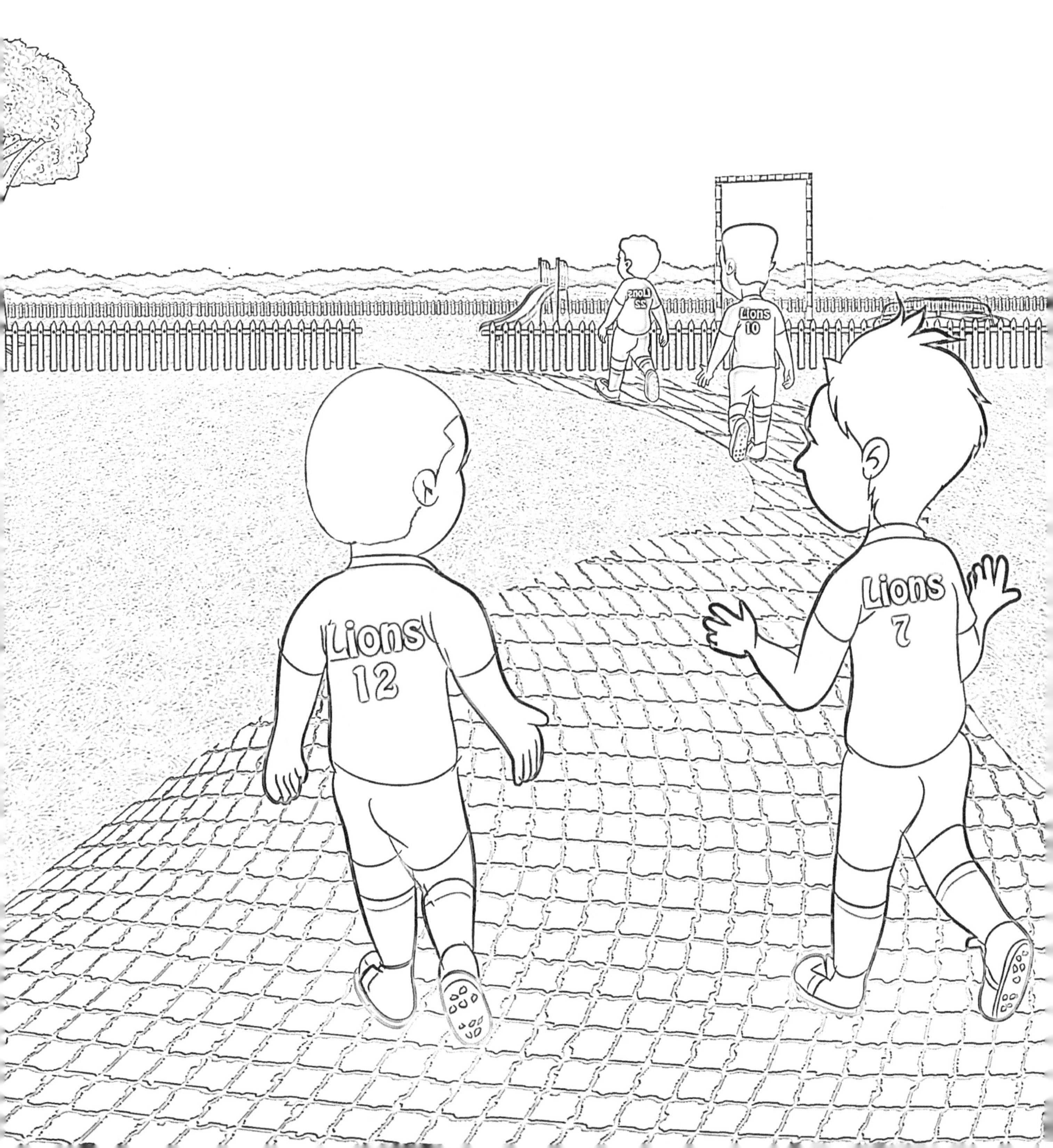

"Let's go to the playground,"
Tebogo says.

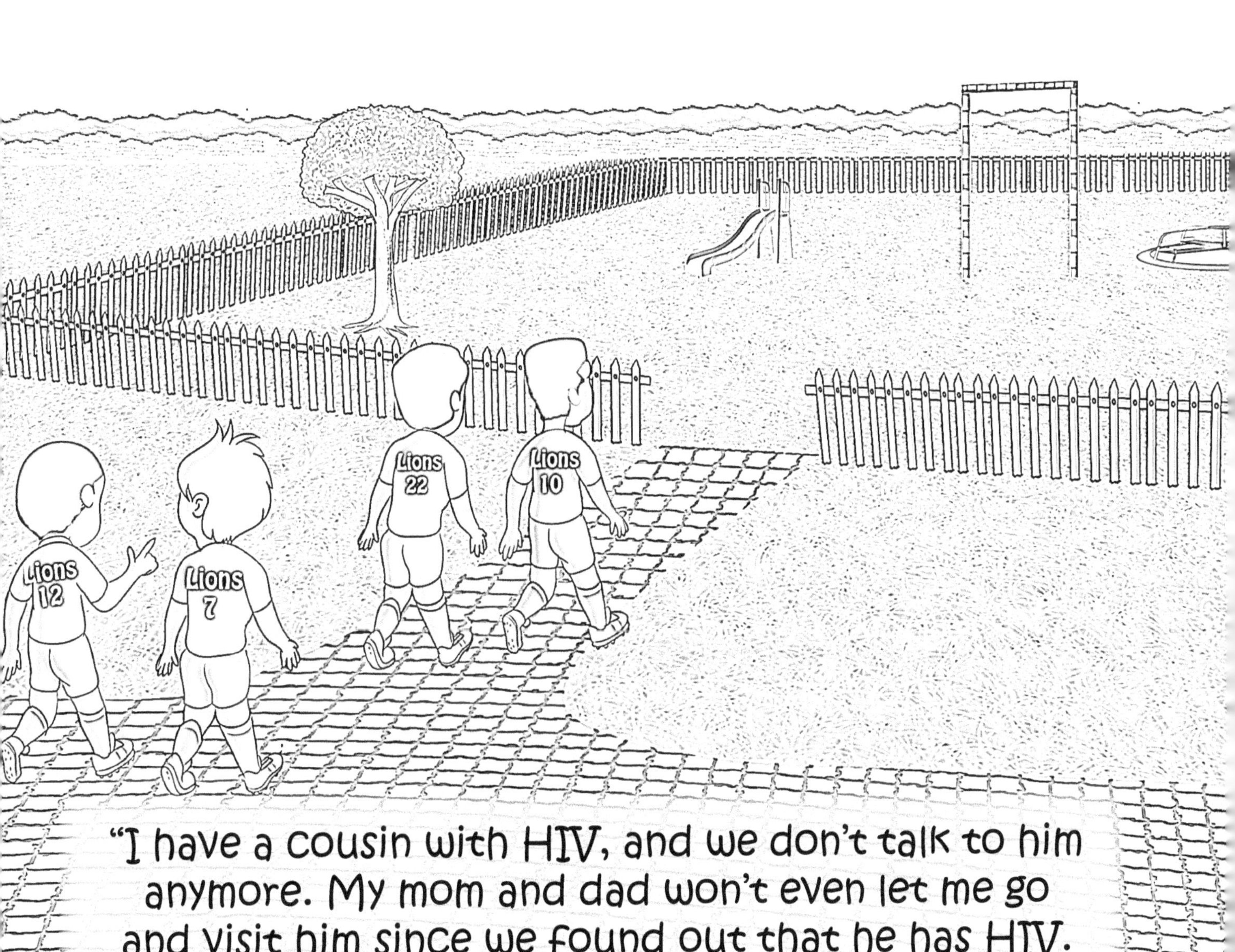

"I have a cousin with HIV, and we don't talk to him anymore. My mom and dad won't even let me go and visit him since we found out that he has HIV. I haven't seen him in a long, long time."
Kasigo said sadly.

"Wow. You can't get HIV from visiting your cousin, nor can you get it from shaking his hand or hugging him." Mpho replied.

"It seems like HIV is kind of hard to get.
All of the ways that I thought you could get it
turned out not to be true.
I now know that you can't get HIV
from touching someone or
shaking someone's hand."
Kagiso said with surprise.

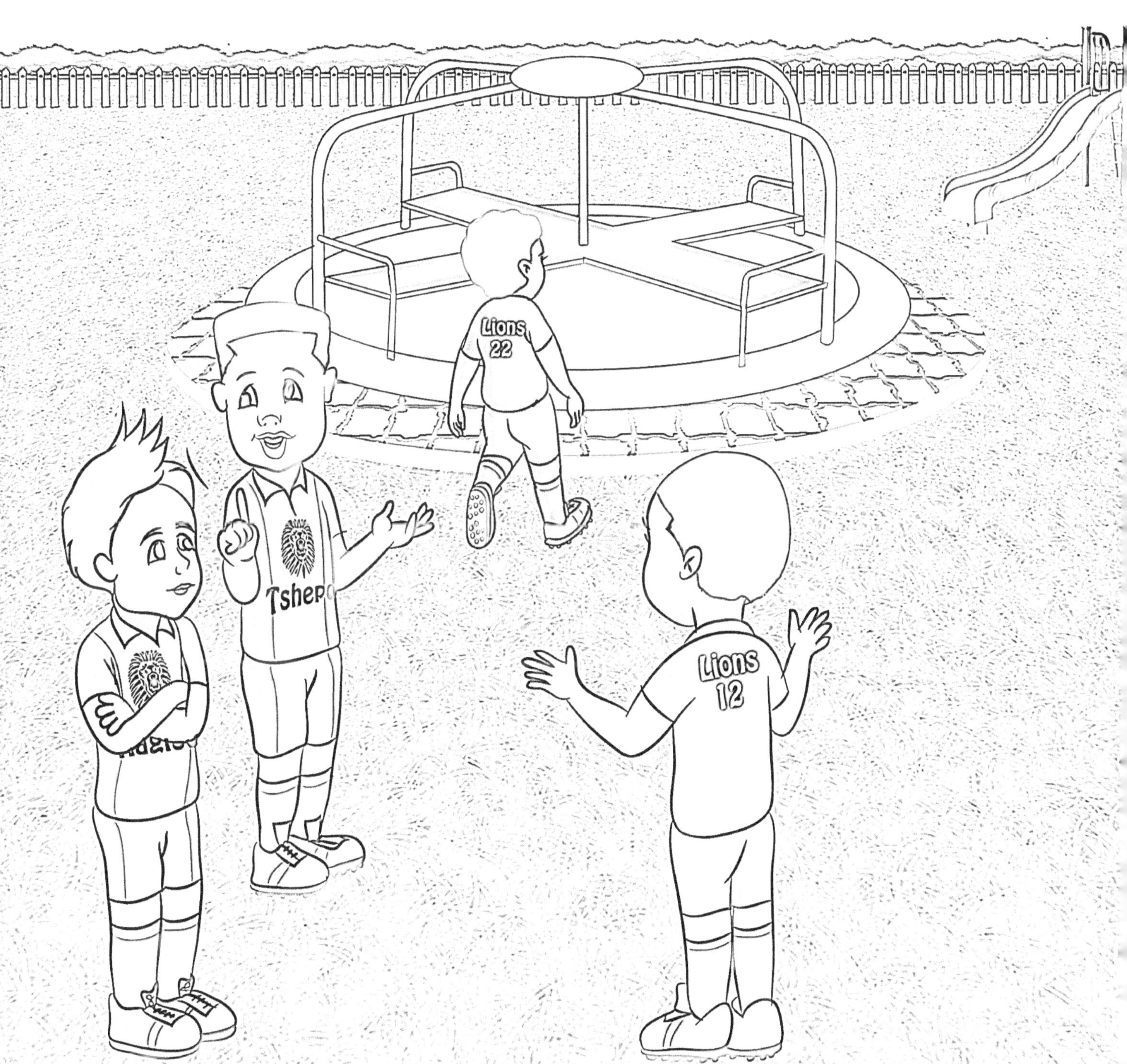

"Don't forget, that Mpho said you can not get HIV
from sharing a room with someone who has HIV or
from visiting someone who has HIV."
Tshepo said with a smile.

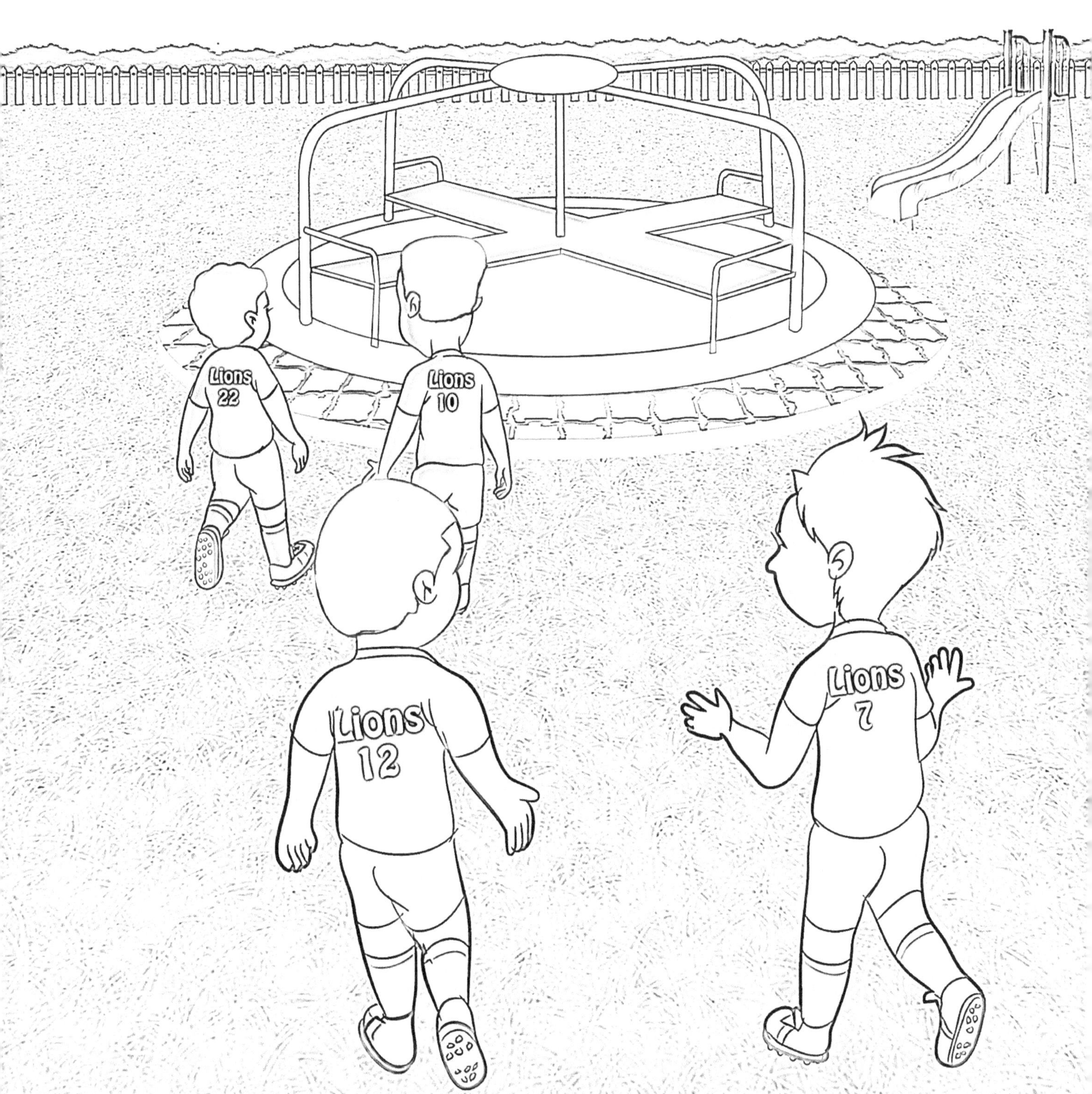

"Oh yeah,
so Mpho, how can you get HIV?" Kagiso asks.

"My family is really nice,
and I'll never get HIV."
Tshepo interrupts saying with confidence.

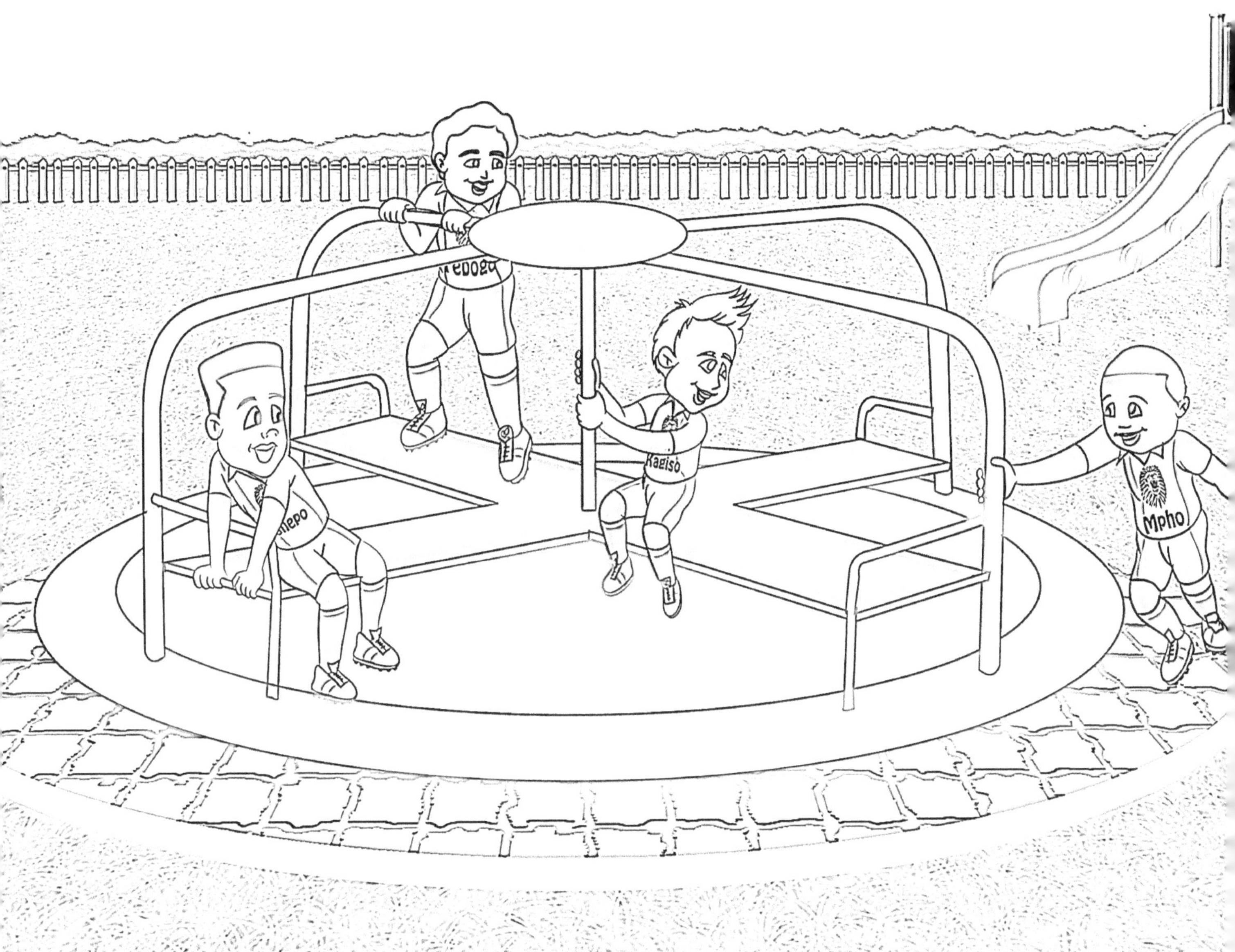

"Don't say that Tshepo. It can happen to anyone.
HIV doesn't look for certain people to infect.
One way to help stop HIV from spreading
is to teach someone else about it." Mpho said.

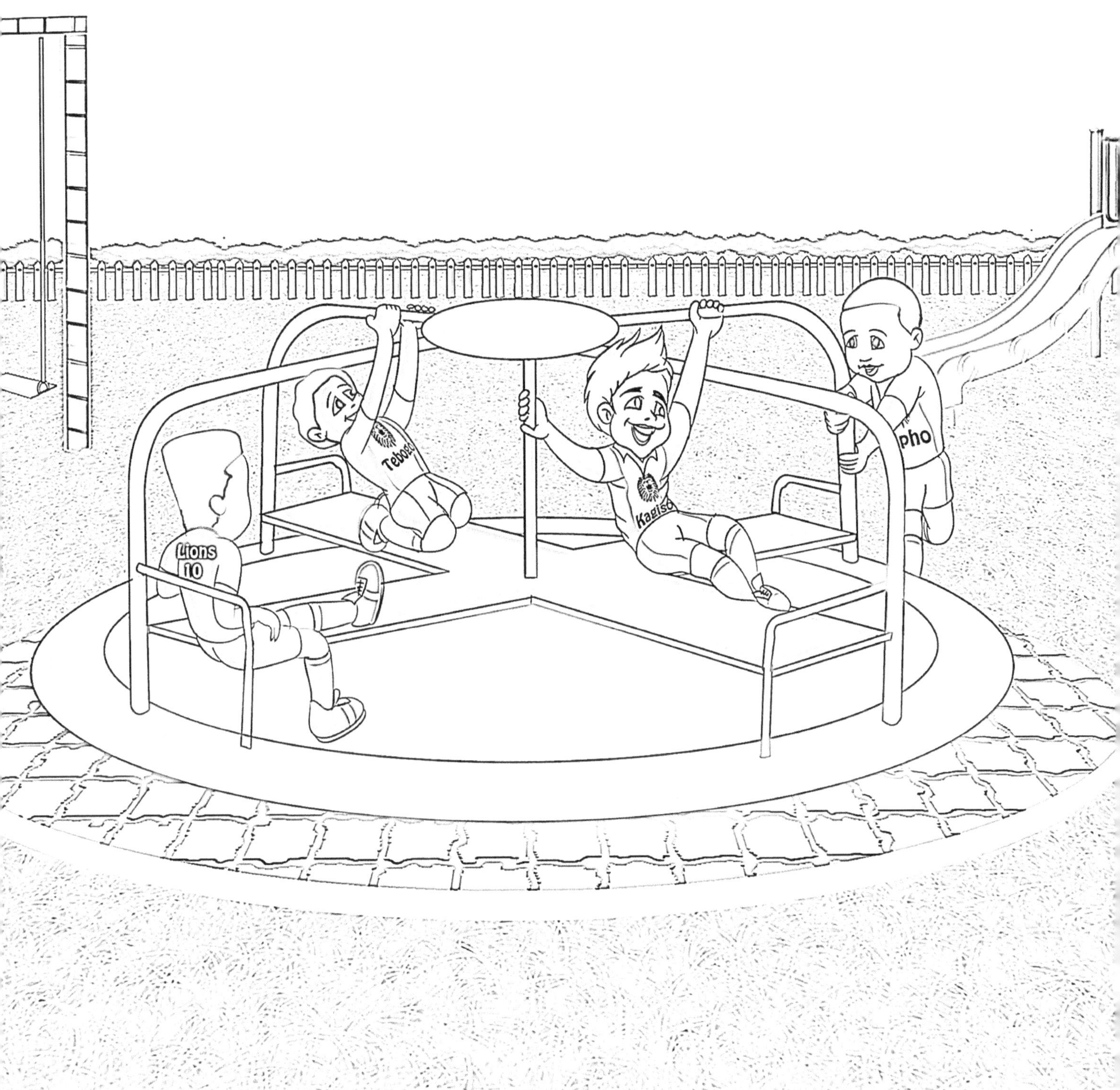

"Okay.
This is so cool for you to tell us all of this Mpho.
You really know a lot about HIV,
and now we do, too." Tshepo said.

"Yeah, thanks for dropping some
knowledge on us Mpho,"
added Tebogo.

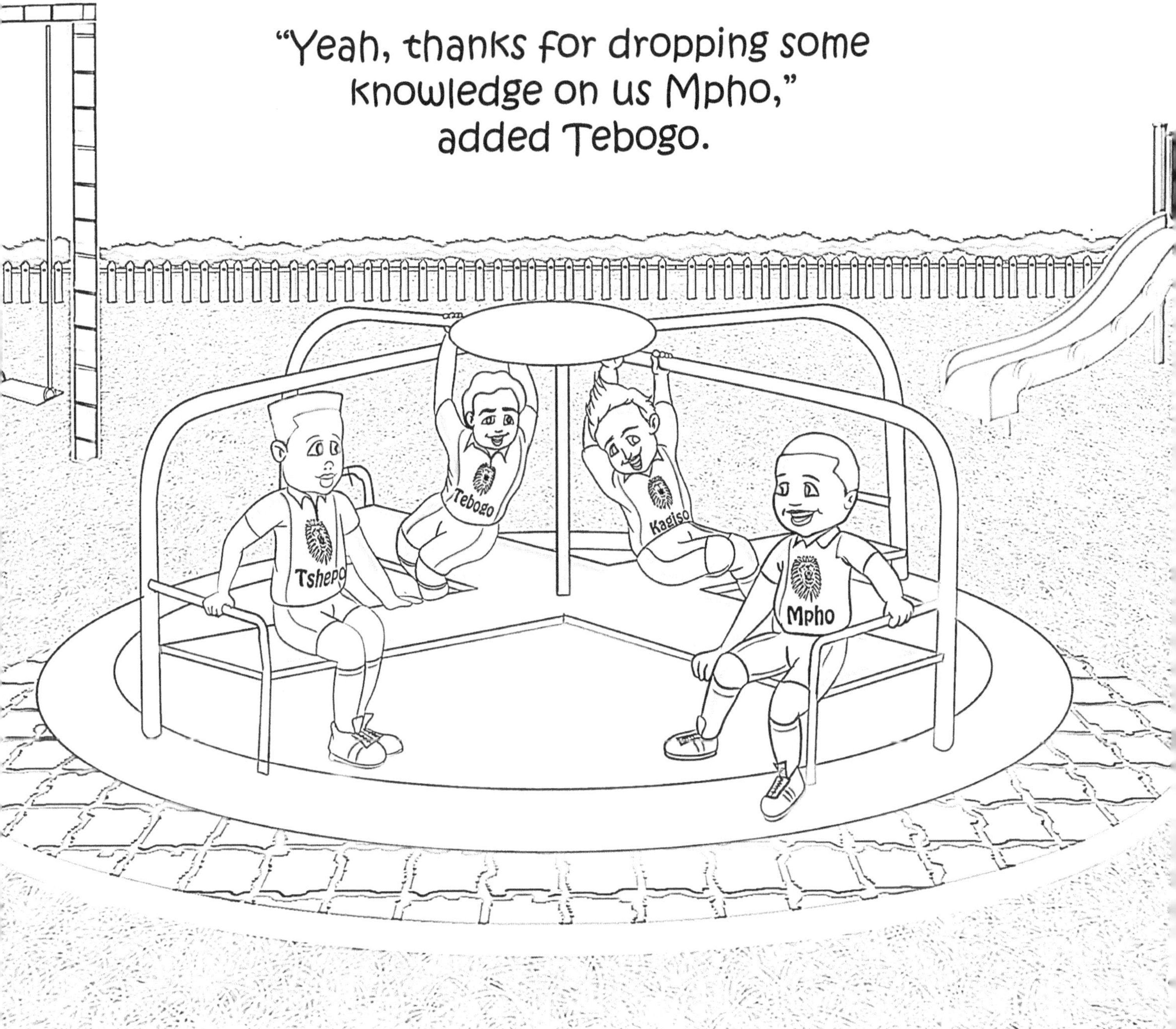

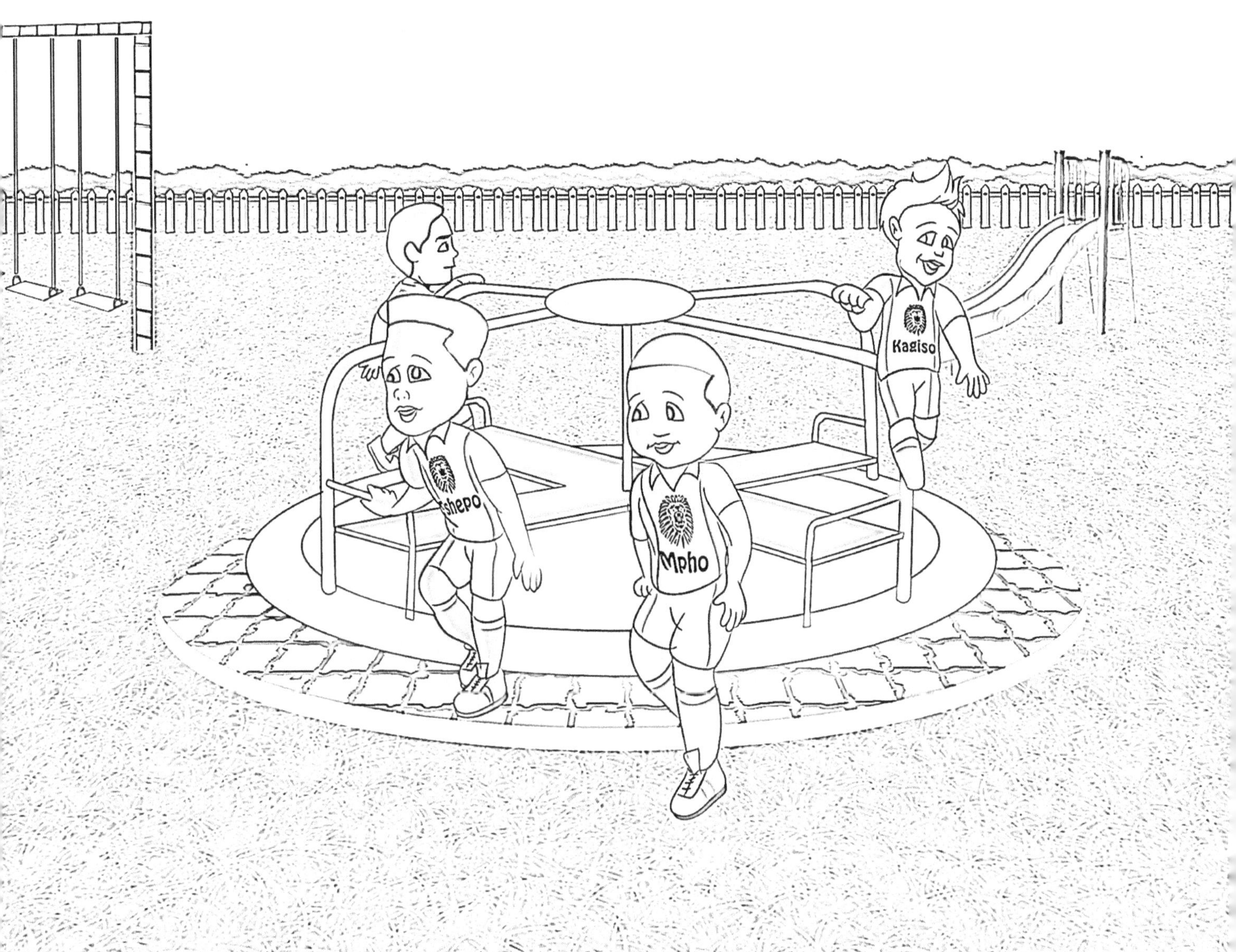

"No problem guys, we are best friends,
and that's what friends are for.
Let's check out the swings before we go home."
Mpho suggests.

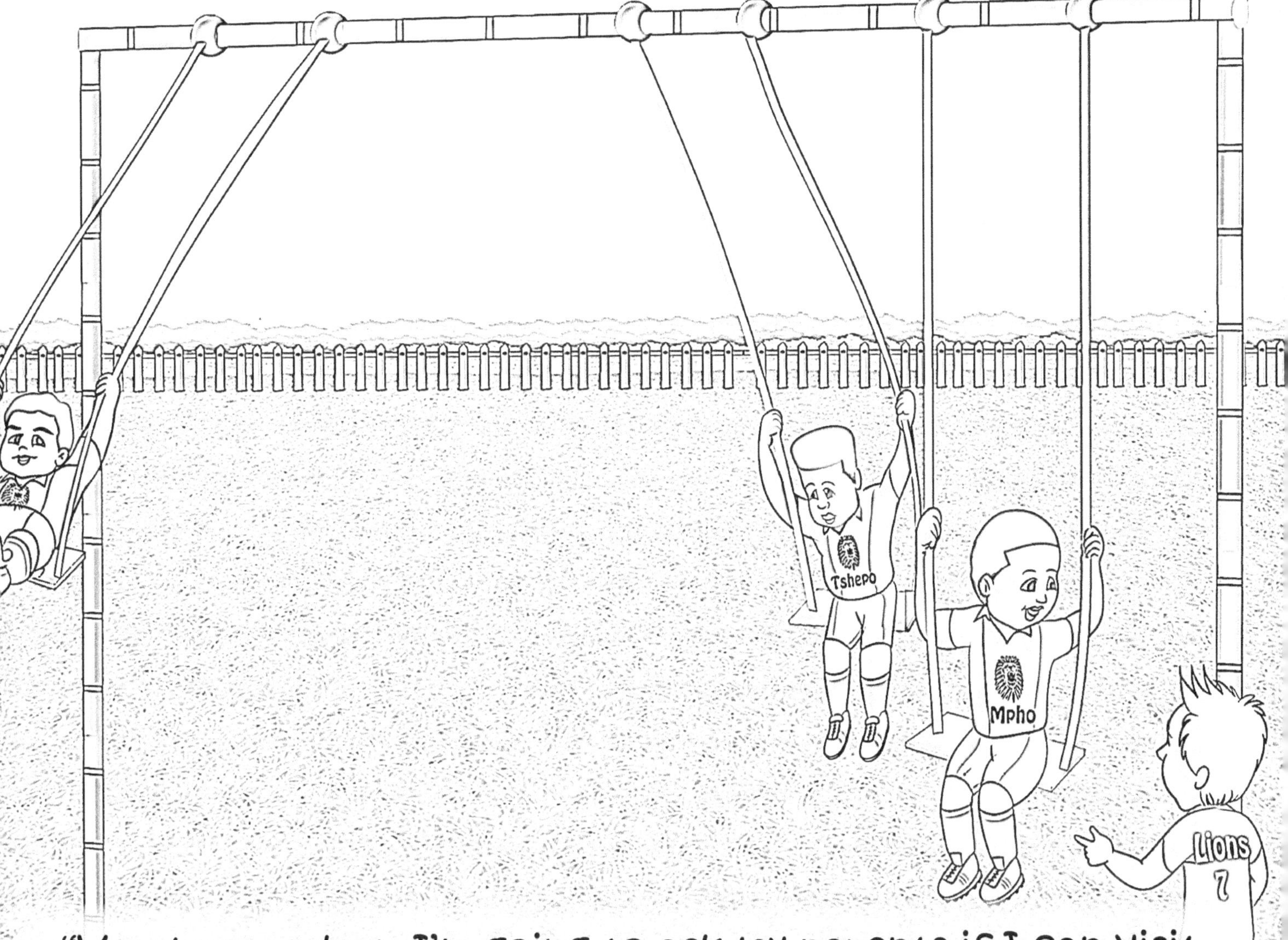

"You know what, I'm going to ask my parents if I can visit my cousin that I told you guys about. As a matter of fact, when I get home, I'm going to tell my mom and dad what I learned, and when I have a chance to visit my cousin, I will be sure to tell him how important it is to take his medicine, because it will keep him healthy." said Kagiso happily.

Mpho smiled and said, "That's good Kagiso. It would likely make your cousin very happy to see you and to know that you learned about HIV."

"Alright Mpho," said Kagiso.

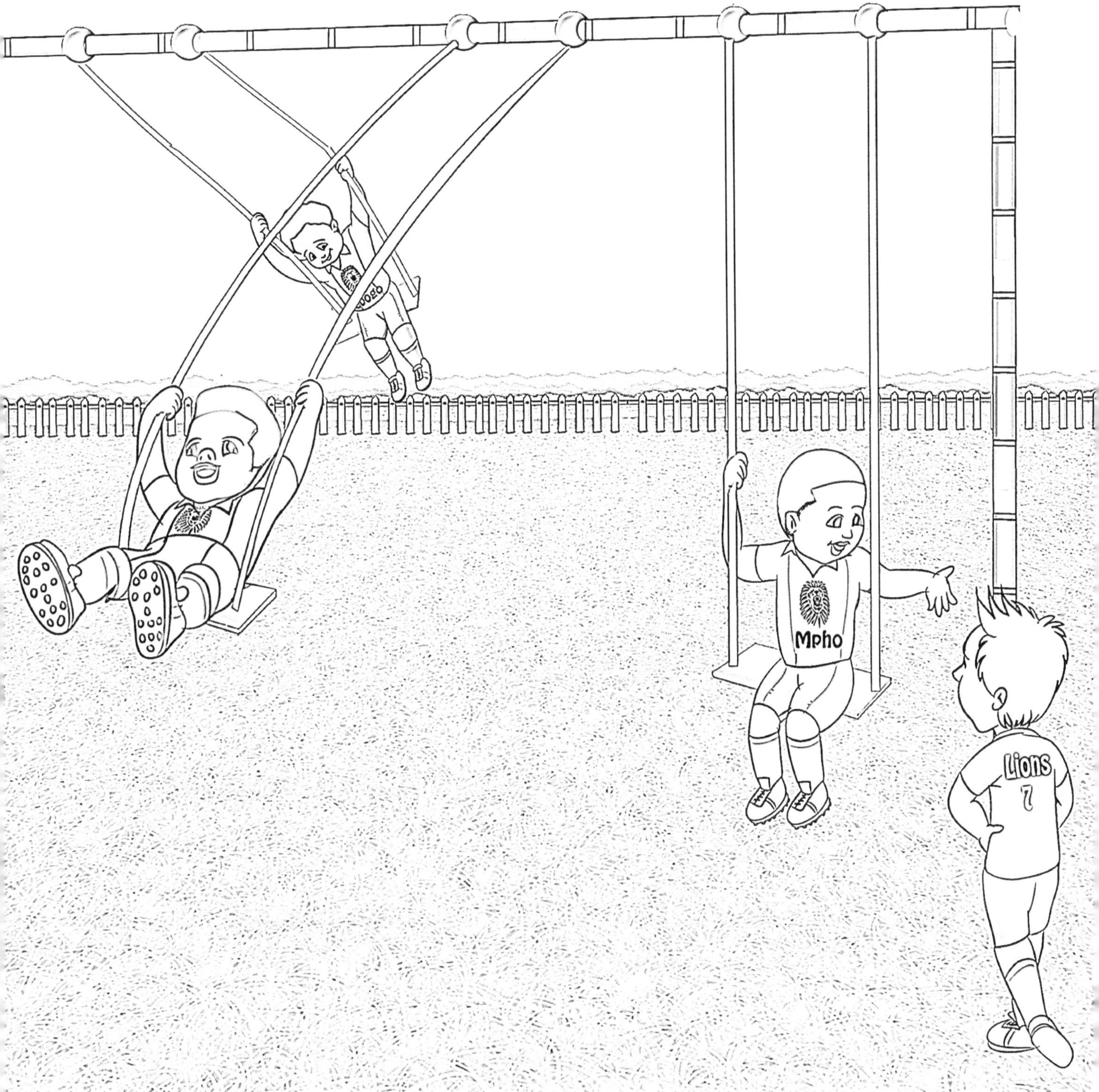

"Hey it's getting kind of late guys,
and my grandmother will start worrying
about me." said Mpho.

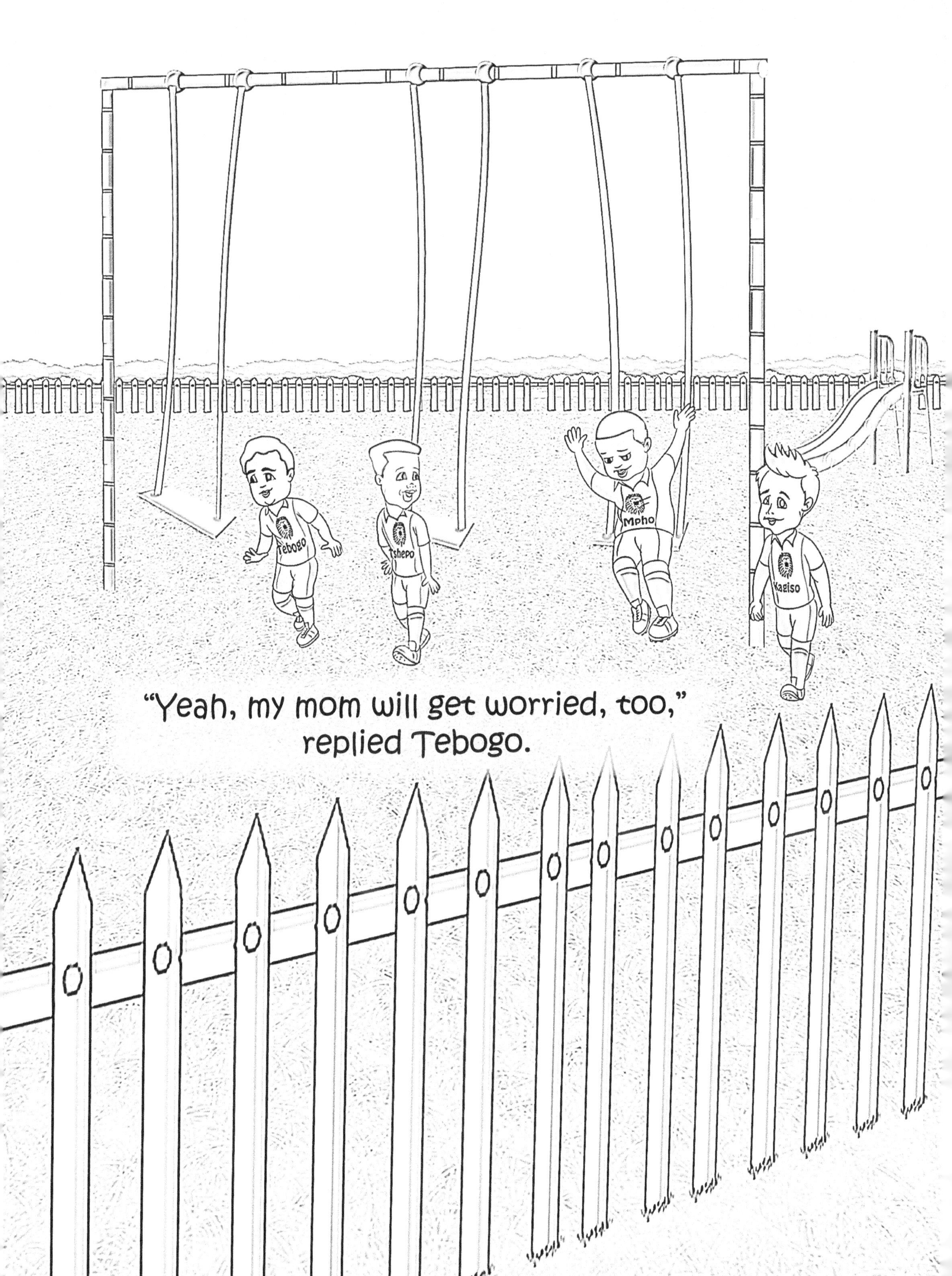

"Yeah, my mom will get worried, too,"
replied Tebogo.

"I'll see you guys at school on Monday."
Mpho says barely able to speak.

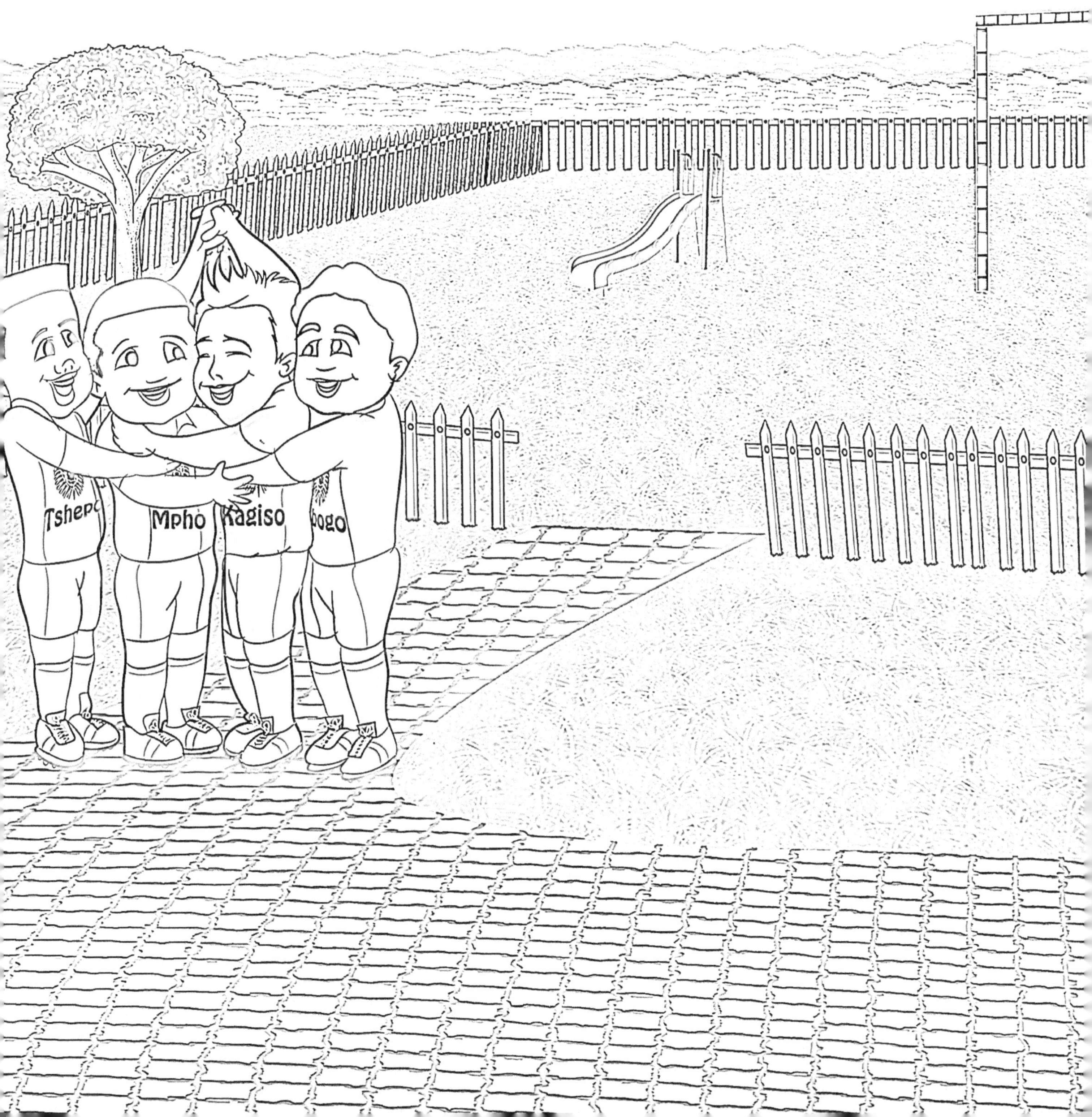

"Bye, guys," said Mpho.
"Bye, Mpho, see you at school on Monday,"
everyone replied.
"Great shot Mpho, we're really proud of you,"
they all said at the same time.

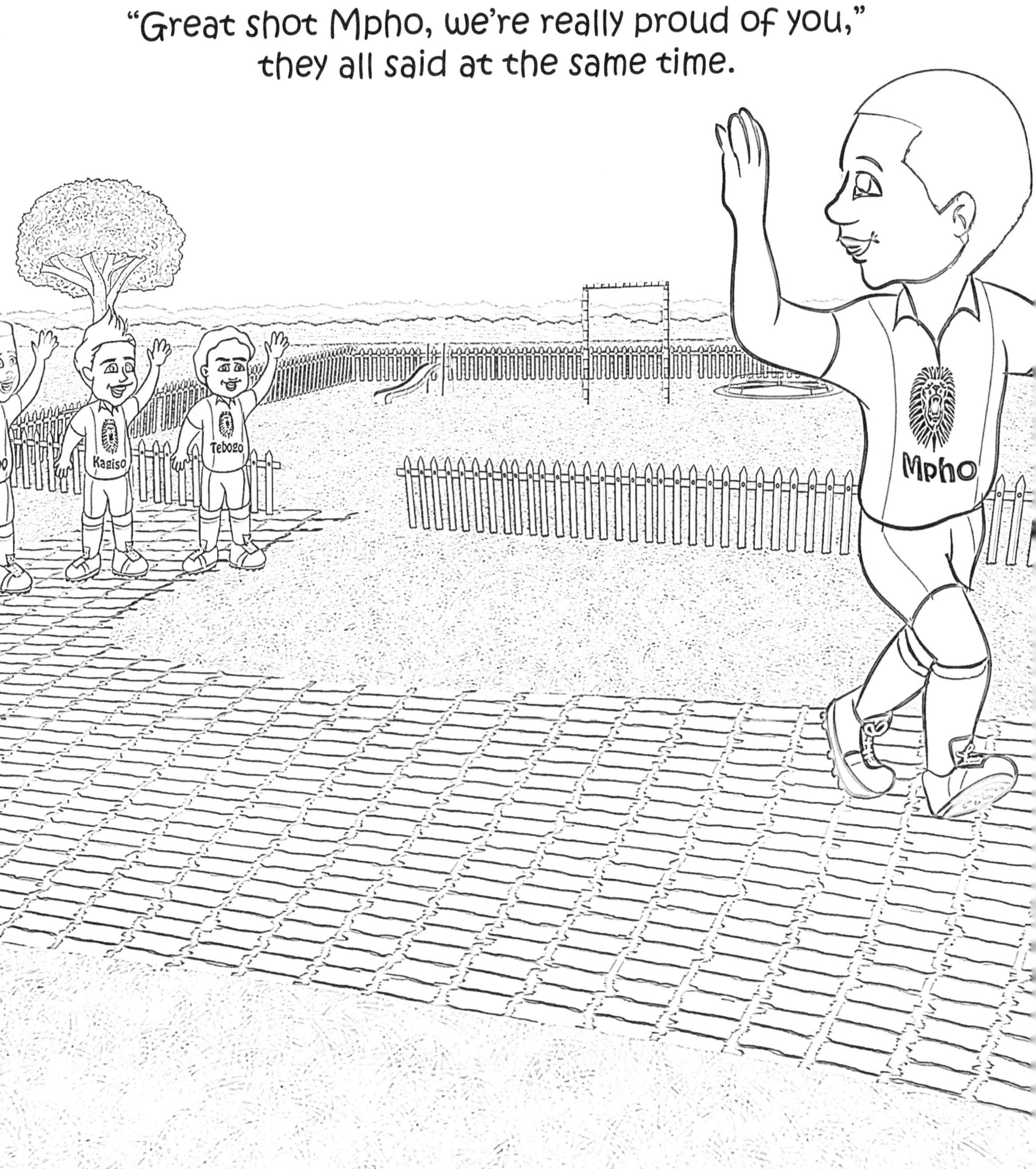

Kagiso
Tebogo
Mpho

LIONS THE CHAMPIONS

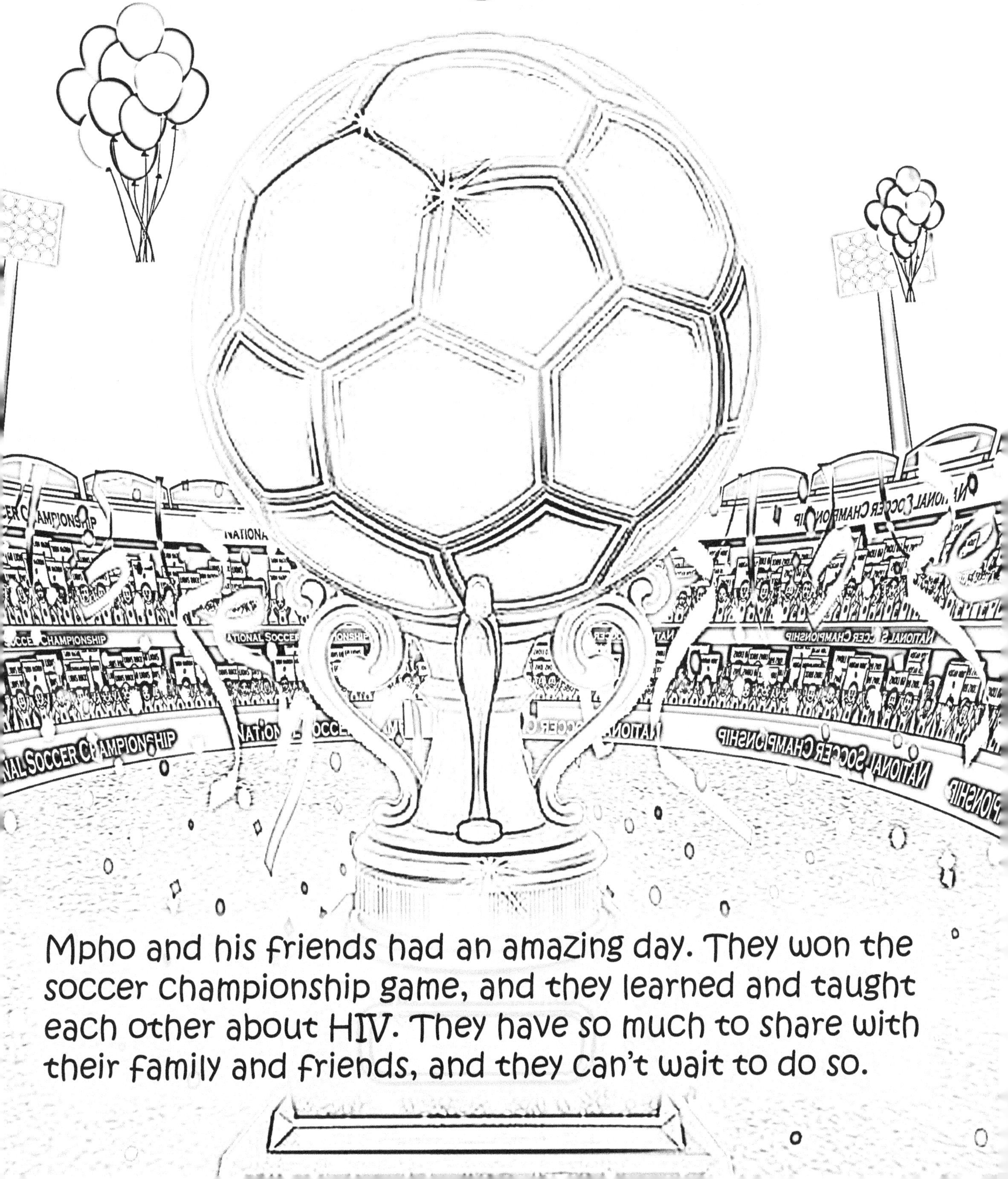

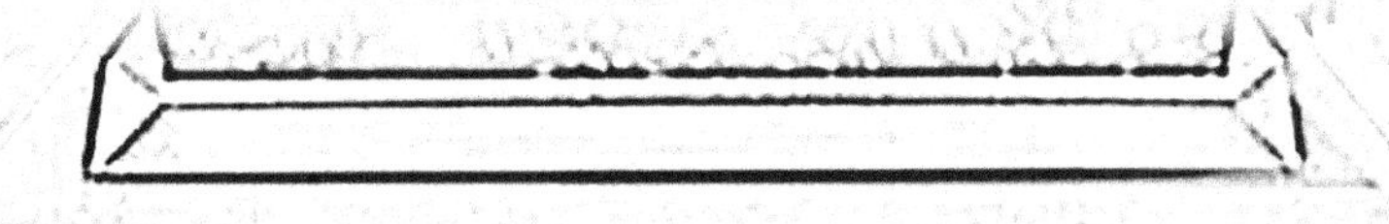

Mpho and his friends had an amazing day. They won the soccer championship game, and they learned and taught each other about HIV. They have so much to share with their family and friends, and they can't wait to do so.

To learn more about HIV/AIDS we encourage you to visit:

Centers for Disease Control and Prevention:

The website of the Centers for Disease Control and Prevention at:

https://www.cdc.gov/hiv/

"CDC works 24/7 to protect America from health, safety and security threats, both foreign and in the U.S. Whether diseases start at home or abroad, are chronic or acute, curable or preventable, human error or deliberate attack, CDC fights disease and supports communities and citizens to do the same.

CDC increases the health security of our nation. As the nation's health protection agency, CDC saves lives and protects people from health threats. To accomplish our mission, CDC conducts critical science and provides health information that protects our nation against expensive and dangerous health threats, and responds when these arise."

AIDSinfo

Visit the website of the US Department of Health and Human services at:

https://aidsinfo.nih.gov/

A service of the US Department of Health and Human Services (HHS), offers access to the latest, federally approved HIV/AIDS medical practice guidelines, HIV treatment and prevention clinical trials, and other research information for health care providers, researchers, people affected by HIV/AIDS, and the general public.

1-800-HIV-0440 (448-0440) | 1-888-480-3739 TTY
1-301-315-2816 (Outside United States)
E-mail at: contactus@aidsinfo.nih.gov

amfAR

Visit their website at:

http://amfar.org/

"Founded in 1985, amfAR is dedicated to ending the global AIDS epidemic through innovative research.

With the freedom and flexibility to respond quickly to emerging areas of scientific promise, amfAR plays a catalytic role in accelerating the pace of HIV/AIDS research and achieving real breakthroughs. Since 1985, amfAR has invested $480 million in its programs and has awarded more than 3,300 grants to research teams worldwide. Through its $100 million Countdown to a Cure for AIDS initiative, amfAR aims to develop the scientific basis for a cure by 2020."

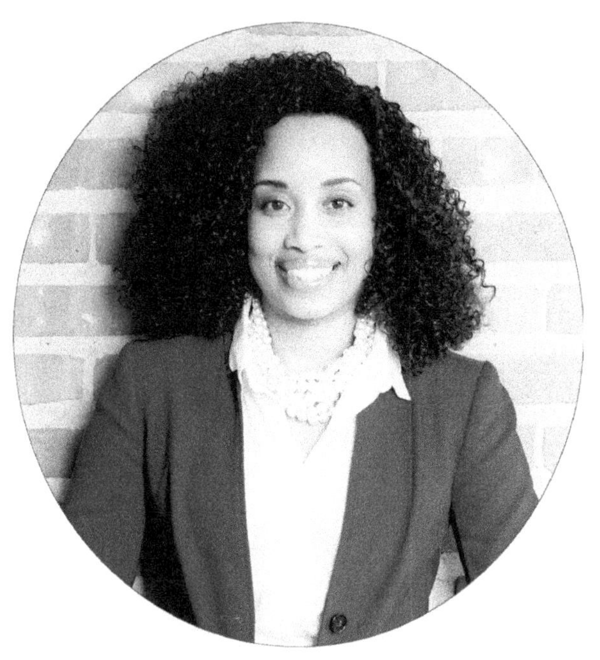

Dr. Wyntrea Cunningham's Biography:

Dr. Cunningham graduated from the Texas A & M University Health Science Center College of Medicine in 2013 and completed residency at the UT Houston Health Science Center/McGovern Medical School. She practices medicine as an Obstetrician and Gynecologist at Specialists in Obstetrics and Gynecology, and is affiliated with The Women's Hospital of Texas in Houston Texas.

Wyntrea was fortunate enough to spend three months in Gaborone, Botswana (Hah-ba-ronay, Bots-wana) conducting research with the Baylor International Pediatric AIDS Initiative (BIPAI). She is passionate about helping dispel the misinformation surrounding HIV/AIDS and after her work in Botswana, Dr. Cunningham decided to write this uplifting, educational and entertaining children's book to help decrease the stigma that is too often associated with HIV/AIDS.

Dr. Cunningham believes that Nelson Mandela was correct when he said,

*"Education is the most powerful weapon
which you can use to change the world."*

The better educated we are about the disease, the less fearful and the more compassionate we can be.

As Plato said,
"Courage is knowing what not to fear."

Mpho's Legacy of Hope is written to dispel the fear and encourage hope and compassion.